COOKING FOR THE
sensitive gut

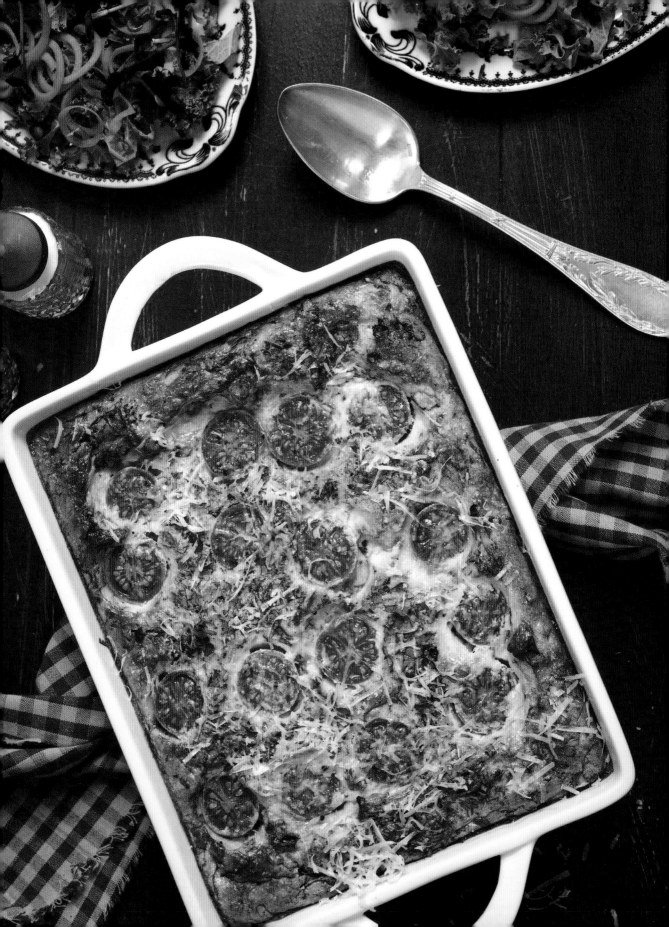

COOKING FOR THE
sensitive gut

DELICIOUS, SOOTHING, HEALTHY RECIPES FOR EVERY DAY
DR JOAN RANSLEY & DR NICK READ

COLLINS & BROWN

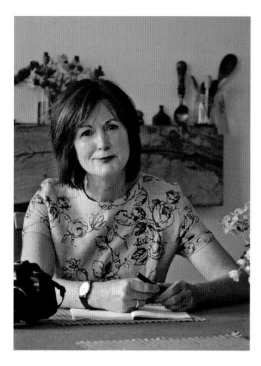

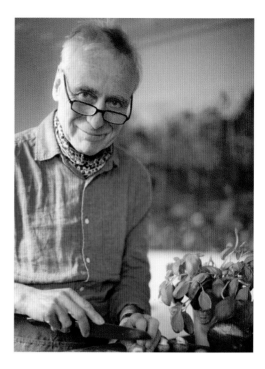

The Authors

Dr Joan Ransley is a freelance nutritionist, food writer and photographer. She is a former lecturer in Human Nutrition at the University of Leeds and holds a Masters degree and PhD in Human Nutrition. Joan is a member of the Guild of Food writers. Joan's food photography has received several awards at the prestigious Pink Lady® Food Photographer of the Year Competition. www.joanransley.co.uk

Dr Nick Read is a gastroenterologist and a psychotherapist. For many years, he was Professor of Human Nutrition and Gastrointestinal Physiology at Sheffield University, before becoming Professor of Integrated Medicine. His popular book, *Sick and Tired: Healing the Illnesses Doctors Cannot Cure*, was published in paperback in August 2006 (Weidenfeld and Nicolson). He was, until 2017, Chair and Medical Adviser for the IBS Network, an independent charity that supports, informs and advises people with irritable bowel syndrome (IBS). He has a long-standing interest in food and cooking. www.nickread.co.uk

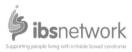

The IBS Network is the UK's national charity for irritable bowel syndrome (IBS). Like many small charities, it punches way above its weight to inform, advise and support people with IBS. It offers a comprehensive web-based IBS Self Care Programme that covers everything anybody would possibly wish to know about IBS, from diagnosis to management of diarrhoea. But it also publishes a monthly newsletter (Relief), a quarterly magazine (*Gut Reaction*), operates a telephone helpline run by IBS nurses, offers advice from IBS professionals by email, coordinates self-help groups and issues 'can't wait' cards for people who need urgent access to a toilet. The charity is supported by a team of IBS patients and health-care professionals. www.theibsnetwork.org

Contents

INTRODUCTION

It is a curious fact that, at a time when those living in the so-called 'developed' world are better nourished than ever before, as many as 30% claim to be intolerant of, or allergic to, the food they eat. Just think back to the last time you had people round for dinner, or went out to a restaurant with friends… How many of them refused to eat something on the menu? Perhaps they were avoiding wheat. Maybe it was milk or dairy. Free-from foods are big business these days, but only about 2% of the adult population has a specific food allergy. The majority have food intolerance.

There is a difference. While food allergies are scientifically measurable, food intolerance is a non-specific sensitivity. Common culprits include fatty foods, chilli or coffee, which all stimulate gut contractions or spasm; coarse wheat bran that directly irritates the gut; and a group of poorly absorbed sugars that can distend a sensitive gut either by drawing in fluid or by being fermented, releasing gases. The latter have been brought together under the term FODMAPs[1] (Fermentable Oligosaccharides, Disaccharides, Monosaccharides and Polyols) and foods containing these sugars include onions, wheat, beetroot, certain fruits and fruit juices and – in some people – milk.

When they go to their doctor, most people with long-standing intolerance to food are diagnosed with irritable bowel syndrome (IBS), a poorly understood disturbance of gastrointestinal sensitivity with no definite cause or specific cure. In a study we carried out together, we found that people who suffered from IBS were sensitive to between 5 and 22 different food components. What's more, their intolerance tended to come and go and was often related to what was happening in their lives. This suggested to us that, in IBS, it is not so much the specific foods that are the problem, but a sensitive gut.

Do you remember when you last spent an afternoon in the sun and then put your top on? Your skin felt as if it were burning. Well, your gut can become sensitive, too. It has sense organs just like the skin; only these respond to stretch and distension, the texture of food, its chemical composition, and any event or situation that upsets the gut. And when these sense organs are over-sensitive, stimulation causes a sensation of pain, fullness or bloating.

IBS does not have to be a life sentence. This book puts you in control of your own illness. Not only will we explain why your gut becomes sensitive, why you can tolerate some foods and not others, and what causes your illness to come and go, but we will also show you how to prepare a huge range of delicious dishes that calm your gut reactions and help you live in confidence with your IBS. What's more, your family will enjoy the recipes, too. Allowing yourself just a little time each day to cook something you love is a form of mindfulness; it relaxes you and gives you control of what you eat. This in itself will help to reduce any anxiety you feel around food, so you can once again look forward to enjoying your meals with confidence.

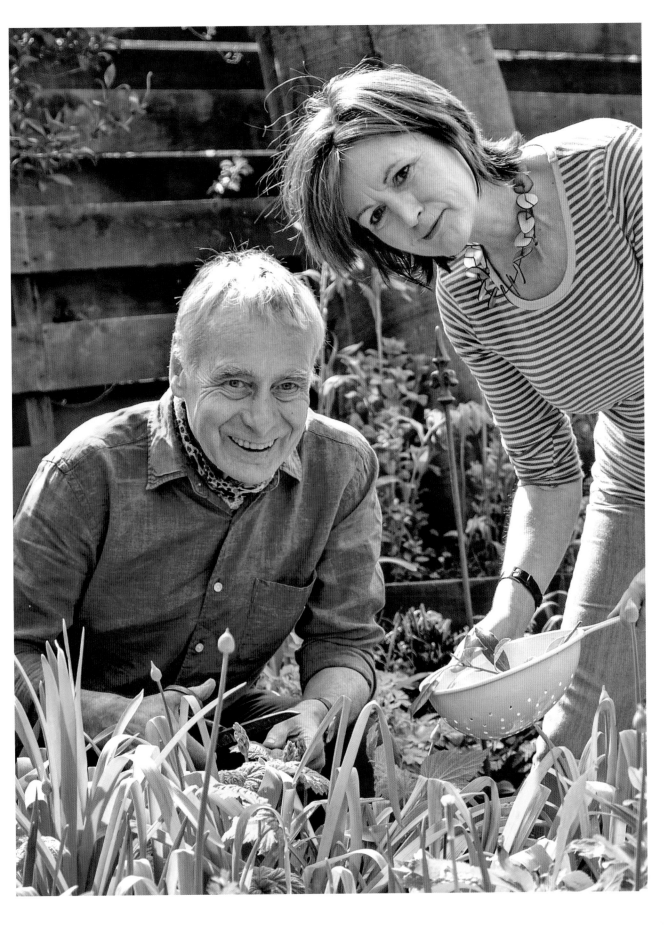

You are what you eat

'Ninety per cent of the diseases known to man are caused by cheap foodstuffs. You are what you eat.'
Victor Lindlahr, 1942

Human beings are omnivores. Our gut evolved when we were hunter-gatherers, feeding on meat, eggs and the roots, leaves, stems, fruits, nuts and seeds of a whole variety of plants… and has probably not changed much since. Nevertheless, within a relatively short span of 10,000 years, the food we eat has altered beyond all recognition.

Stable communities were built on the husbandry of animals, which produced milk as well as meat, and the cultivation of grasses to create cereals that could be ground into flour. We learned how to preserve and store food to feed us over winter or in times of famine. Cooking changed the consistency and palatability of foods, making them easier to digest and more appetising. Spices improved their flavour and assisted digestion. Growing crops worldwide on an industrial scale has meant that we no longer rely on seasonal produce, but can buy any food we want from our local supermarket.

This exciting new culinary world comes at a cost. We still have the digestive system of a Neolithic hunter-gatherer, not always able to cope with the sheer volume and variety of the highly processed food that we eat today.

For example, as soon as they are weaned, 80% of people in the world lose the enzyme that enables them to digest lactose (milk sugar), rendering them potentially intolerant to dairy products. Between 14 and 60% of people with IBS report that they are sensitive to cultivars of wheat, the staple food of 35% of the world's population. Fructose, which is largely responsible for the sweetness of many fruits, is only slowly absorbed in the small intestine. The excess is rapidly fermented in the colon, which might explain why fruits and concentrated fruit juices can upset so many of us.

Many of the vegetables and fruits we eat contain complex starches and sugars that we cannot digest. Cows exist mainly on grass, but they have a 40-gallon fermenter for a stomach. Lacking their prodigious capabilities, we and our sensitive guts often struggle to cope with cereals, fruits and vegetables.

And although our gut may have evolved to digest and absorb gargantuan quantities of fat – to supply the energy to last through the winter or times of famine – an overabundance of rich and fatty foods all year round has contributed to a disastrous epidemic of obesity and related diseases.

But before we consider why the gut may have become so sensitive, we need to understand how it works.

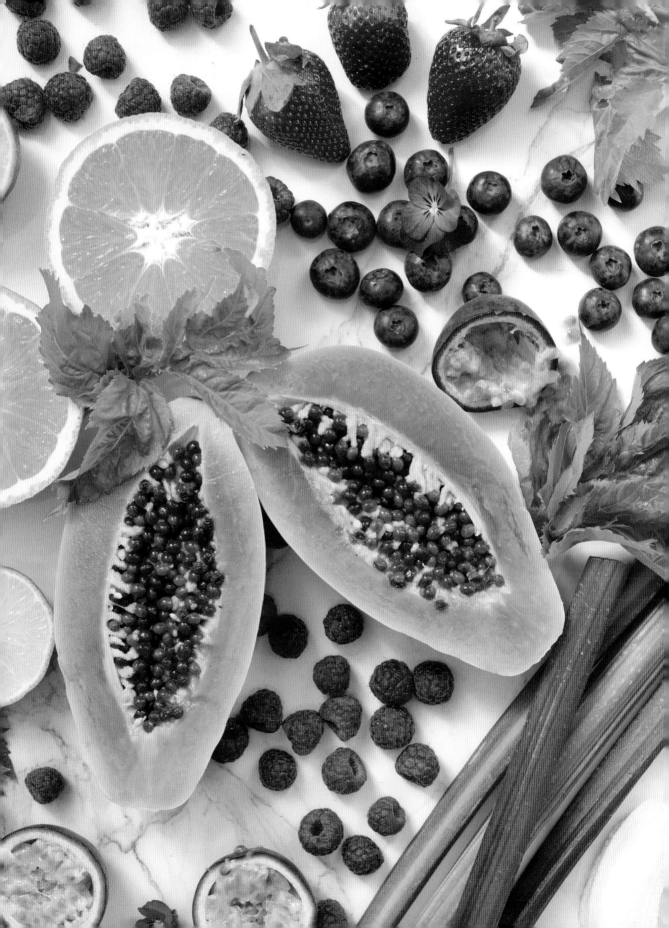

How the gut works

We have, coiled inside our abdomen, a food processor that is customised to everything we eat. The gut is a tube, 7–10 metres (20–30 feet) long, a chopper, mixer, digester, extractor and salvage system in one, an industrious conveyer belt that dismantles food to its fundamental components and absorbs these for energy, growth, defence, repair and all the processes that keep the body healthy and functional.

Humans do not eat continuously, as do cattle or sheep, which need to process enormous quantities of grass to obtain enough energy for survival. Neither do we eat like large carnivores, such as lions, that binge after a kill, then rest up for a few days before hunting again. Nevertheless, we carry the imprints of both those evolutionary lifestyles in the design of our gut. Our foregut (stomach, gall bladder, pancreas and small intestine) is more like that of a carnivore, while our hindgut is specialised for the digestion of plant material like that of a horse. So from an evolutionary perspective, we are neither grazers nor bingers – although some may adopt those lifestyles; we are batch feeders.

Every day most of us process about 2 kg (4 lb) of solid food and 1.5 litres (2½ pints) of fluid in three meals, each separated by gaps of about four hours. As food is eaten, solids are broken up by chewing, lubricated with saliva, and moulded by the tongue and the palate into small soft lumps. These are swallowed and propelled into the stomach by the strong peristaltic contractions of the oesophagus.

The stomach is a muscular bag that can hold as much as 3 litres (5 pints). It secretes a mixture of quite strong hydrochloric acid (pH 1) and peptic enzymes, which soften the collagen fibres that hold meat together and start to digest the protein. As digestion proceeds, regular contractions advance down the conical gastric antrum like the incoming tide, pushing the softening food, which squirts back through the aperture of the advancing wave. This churns the food, dispersing the fat into an emulsion with protein, and converting the whole meal into an acidic slurry which is propelled in spurts through a narrow outlet called the pylorus into the duodenum.

It takes two to four hours for a meal to empty from the stomach. Large meals, more viscous foods and those that are rich in fat are emptied more slowly. As the liquefied meal passes through the duodenum, bile and chemical enzymes are added to continue the process of digestion of protein, fat and starch into components that are small enough to be conveyed across the cells lining the small intestine into the blood. Protein is disintegrated into small peptides and amino acids. Fat is broken into glycerol and fatty acids. Starch is dismantled into glucose.

The carbohydrate part of the diet contains some components that are poorly absorbed in the small intestine, so go on to be salvaged in the colon by fermentation. These include lactose (milk sugar), fructose, sugar alcohols (polyols) and the larger more complex sugars (fructans and galactans) that exist in many vegetables and cereals.

In healthy people eating a balanced diet, about 90% of the energy and nutrients from food is absorbed in the small intestine, leaving about 1.5 litres (2½ pints) of bitter yellow slurry to be propelled into the colon. But there is considerable variation in the volume of this effluent. An abnormally rapid passage through the small intestine limits time for absorption to take place and increases the amount of effluent. Both food and mood can exert a profound effect on small bowel transit time. Foods that contain a lot of fruits and fruit juices tend to accelerate transit, while fats slow it down. Stress, excitability and any cause of intestinal irritation or sensitivity can speed things up. Rapid transit limits the absorption of most foods, dumping large amounts of semi-digested residues – plus irritant bile acid – into an already sensitive colon.

COLONIC SALVAGE

Until recently the colon was viewed as the dark continent of the human body, a Stygian swamp, packed full of a trillion wriggling, squirming, teeming organisms: bacteria, fungi and viruses. The discovery of the 'microbiome', the collective term for all the micro-organisms in our colon, has been like finding a new organ in the body; it is a metabolic powerhouse that can break down almost any organic substance and has a diversity of function far greater than that of the liver. This has enormous implications for our nutrition, health and wellbeing.

Much of whatever remains after passage through the small intestine is salvaged in the colon by bacterial fermentation, which can take two days or more. This includes many indigestible components of the plants we eat, collectively known as dietary fibre, a combination of resistant starches and non-starch polysaccharides. Smaller, less complex carbohydrates may also be salvaged in the colon. These include fructo-oligosaccharides (FOS) that are prevalent in onions, garlic, leeks, chicory roots, artichokes, beetroots, brassicas (cabbages, broccoli or sprouts) and asparagus, as well as in wheat and barley; and also galacto-oligosaccharides (GOS), which occur in lentils, chickpeas and beans. Unabsorbed lactose and fructose may also be salvaged in the colon.

Fermentation of carbohydrate releases quantities of odourless gases – hydrogen, carbon dioxide and methane. An average of about 2 litres of gas is produced by a normal person every day, though some people can produce considerably more depending on the nature of the unabsorbed sugars or starches and the composition of the bacteria in the colon. The smaller the unabsorbed sugar or starch molecule, the more rapidly the gas is produced. Gas distends the colon, blowing it up like a balloon and, if the gut is already sensitive, this produces bloating, pain and flatulence. The gases may also affect bowel habit. Methane, for example, may cause constipation.

Under normal circumstances, colonic salvage stimulates the extraction of salt and water, leaving a solid plug of about 200 g/7 oz of bacteria and indigestible fibre, which is evacuated. Colonic salvage can fail if the bacterial populations in the colon are depleted, or if there is a flood of unabsorbed effluent from the small intestine, due to rapid small bowel transit or the retention of fluid by incompletely absorbed lactose, fructose or polyols. When small bowel transit is rapid, fats and bile acids may also escape absorption in the small intestine and irritate the colon inducing peristalsis and fluid secretion. Under those conditions, the contents may be voided as diarrhoea.

The little brain in the gut

The gut has its own brain, consisting of an extensive network of nerve cells and interconnecting fibres. This has all the main features of a true brain: a variety of sense organs that detect changes in its content; a web of connections that integrate signals from these sensors; and a system of 'effectors' that respond to stimulation by altering contractile activity, absorption and secretion, sensation and immune function. Feedback via the gut-brain coordinates the rate of digestion with the delivery of food from the stomach, optimises transit through the small intestine and adjusts absorption and secretion. And, like the brain in your head, the gut-brain has a memory. Infection and trauma can make it more sensitive and responsive to both food and mood. So our gut-brain might be regarded as having its own personality, determined by its responses to a unique life experience.

Emotions and the gut

'Our digestions, going peacefully and sacredly onwards. That is the source of all poetry. The most poetical thing in the world is not being sick.'
GK Chesterton, *The Man who was Thursday*

Big cats, lions and tigers rest for several days after a kill; hunting dogs and wolves do the same. If their digestive torpor is interrupted, they will often vomit before running away. Other species evacuate their bowels if they are disturbed or frightened. Greylag geese eat grass, which is fermented in twin sacs, or *caeci*, which branch off from their large intestine. Konrad Lorenz, pioneer of animal behaviour, tells how he once alarmed the pet geese in his study, whereupon they evacuated their twin *caeci* all over his priceless Persian rug[2].

Our digestions can behave in a similar way. If we have an argument during a meal, if we perform vigorous exercise too soon after eating, or even if we just *think* about a food we don't like, we can get indigestion, feel sick or have to find a lavatory. These reactions are mediated by the autonomic nervous system.

The autonomic (or automatic) nervous system regulates arousal throughout the body for the purposes of survival. There are two components; the sympathetic and the parasympathetic. The sympathetic nervous system uses adrenaline and noradrenaline to prepare the body for hunting, defence or escape (fight or flight). The parasympathetic nervous system facilitates functions of growth, restoration and conservation, such as digestion, sleep, healing and pregnancy. When we are functioning normally, these two systems work together to keep us in an optimal state of engagement with our environment and ourselves, enabling digestion when the body is resting and inhibiting the activity of the gut when the body needs to divert resources to deal with threats.

But, despite our best intentions, we rarely live balanced, restful lives. There are too many calls on our time. All too often, we 'eat on the hoof', rushing to the next appointment or struggling to meet deadlines. This creates a conflict in the gut; the tense, sensitive sympathetic system trying to close it down, while the parasympathetic is still trying to relax and digest lunch. So the beleaguered gut draws attention to its conflict by becoming bloated, painful, blocked up or – in *extremis* – by evacuating its contents like Lorenz's geese.

It is the autonomic nervous system that connects the gut to the brain. Ten times as many nerve fibres transmit information to the brain about the state of the gut than carry instructions to the gut from the brain. This allows whatever is happening in the gut to modulate our behaviour. For example, the presence of fat in the gut after a meal can make us sleepy; sugar accelerates heart rate and makes us feel energetic; irritants or toxins cause nausea, vomiting or diarrhoea. Information from the gut informs us when to rest, eat or stop eating, when to be sick and when to go to the loo.

Most parasympathetic nerves from the gut are connected to the base of the brain. These modulate appetite, hunger and fullness and encourage digestion and absorption by stimulating digestive secretions, intestinal movements and blood flow. Parasympathetic fibres from the end of the gut enter the lowest part of the spinal cord and facilitate colonic movements and defaecation.

The sympathetic nervous system is a major component of our alarm system. So events that frighten us or make us angry stimulate 'gut reactions', while all too often the thinking parts of the brain – the cognitive frontal lobes – go off-line until we can find the space to reconnect and decide what to do. If we fail to reconnect and process what has happened, then we may be left with a gut that is hyper-sensitive and over-reacts to anything that reminds it of those events, as well as to what we eat.

If the gut is injured, inflamed, obstructed or sensitised by stress or trauma, uncomfortable sensations from the gut travel up the same sympathetic nerve routes that transmit sensation from the skin, which explains why pain from different regions of the gut are 'referred' to different areas on the body surface. Visceral pain sets up an alarm reaction, which blocks rational thought and adds a dominant emotional component to the pain.

First line of defence

The gut is the body's most vulnerable line of defence against invasion by foreign organisms or toxic substances. Our food consists of an enormous variety of different chemicals; some, such as alcohol, are quite toxic. It also contains bacteria, fungi, viruses… and even a few insects. Every spoonful we eat is smothered in bugs. Most are relatively harmless, but it's easy to pick up bacteria that cause gastroenteritis from food that has been allowed to cool uncovered, or from utensils, surfaces, toilets and swimming pools.

Our bodies have a well-organised system of defence. Our major senses – vision, smell and taste – inform us if food is fresh and good to eat; the acidic environment of our stomach disinfects our food; bile also contains antibacterial substances; and parts of the intestine recognise the most common dangers and secrete antibodies like a layer of fire-fighting foam, to destroy, detoxify and immobilise them.

A thin red line of cells, just one cell thick, is all that lies between the contents of our gut and the rest of our body. But this is no passive barrier, it is the most heavily fortified defence system in the body. Not only is it reinforced by the big guns of the gut immune system – the largest concentration of immune cells in the body – it is also helped by a highly sophisticated communication network that contains more nerve cells than the brain and can respond to attack at a moment's notice. And this whole defensive array is primed and assisted by the overwhelming concentration of partisans in the colonic microbiome, many of which secrete antibacterial chemicals.

The vast colonies of bacteria that live in our colon are, for the most part, beneficial. Since these immigrants have been there since the beginning, the gut immune system has developed a comfortable state of tolerance and essentially lets them do their thing with little interference. These peaceful long-term residents safeguard us against invasion from more aggressive species by creating an environment that discourages their growth and priming the immune system to be vigilant to their presence. If we did not have such a diverse, multicultural microbiome, our gut immune system would be under a near-constant state of siege, hypersensitive and reacting to everything as if it were a threat.

But as anybody who has made their own wine, or has made bread from sourdough (see page 54), knows, it takes time and specific conditions for a beneficial community of bacteria to become established and work together effectively and in harmony. Unfortunately, the way we lead our lives can all too easily threaten this delicate symbiosis. Powerful antibiotics, prescribed to fight off infections, can decimate the colonic microbiome. Gut infections may lead to diarrhoea, flushing the good bugs out. Our refined diet may deplete the microbiome of essential energy and nutrients. Too much alcohol encourages the growth of harmful bacteria that break it down, increasing the permeability of the gut to toxins and causing inflammation. Or psychological stress may threaten the delicate colonic ecosystem by altering delivery from the small intestine, stimulating contractile activity and compromising immune function.

There is evidence that the microbiome is depleted and destabilised in people with IBS. This could well render the colon more permeable and vulnerable to attack, putting its defences into a state of high alert with mild inflammation and increased sensitivity. Moreover, the release of chemical transmitters from inflammatory cells will stimulate the nerves in the gut and their connections with the brain, changing our mood, making us tired, affecting the way we think and causing alterations in function not only in the gut but throughout the body.

And despite all the body's defence systems, the guerrilla forces of salmonella, shigella, campylobacter or norovirus can occasionally invade the gut wall and stimulate the immune system to counterattack.

Once invasion takes place, white cells gather at the site of the breaches and attempt to destroy the invaders, while immune cells either annihilate the attackers or immobilise them with antibodies. Meanwhile, the inflamed gut attempts to get rid of the danger with vomiting and diarrhoea. But this isn't always the end of it. In about 15% of cases, the traumatised gut remembers the assault, and the immune system remains in a state of hyper-vigilance and mild inflammation, hyper-sensitive to the risk of further attack and even to foods that stimulate the gut.

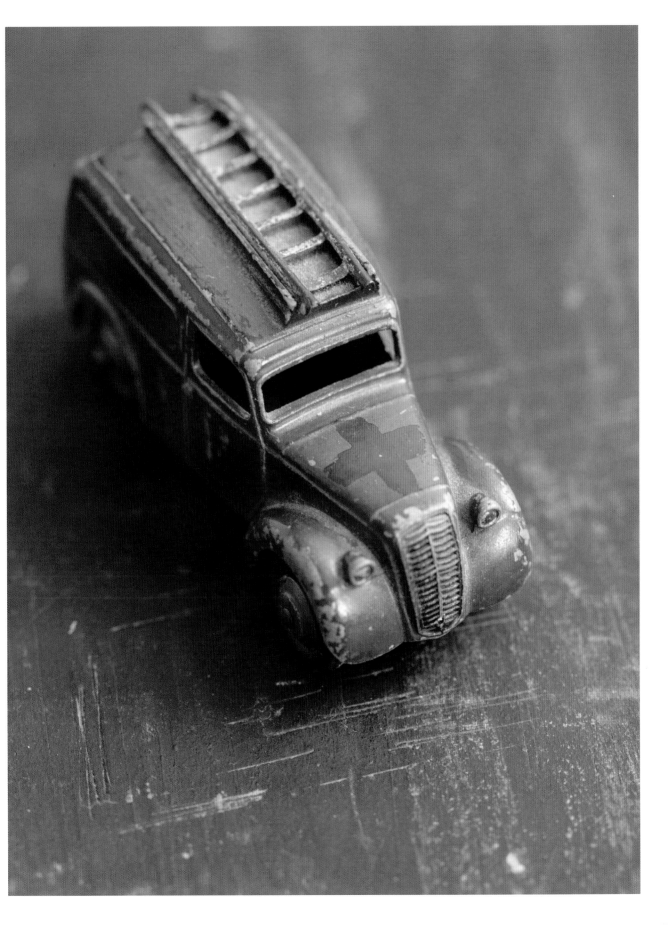

What is a sensitive gut?

More an exaggerated state of arousal than a diagnosis, a sensitive gut over-reacts to changes in diet and life situations with symptoms of abdominal discomfort and gut reactions, such as vomiting, diarrhoea, constipation or abdominal distension. This might be regarded as the character of a person's gut, the visceral expression of the individual. So depending on who you are, your personal history, how you feel and what you have eaten, a sensitive gut can make you feel sick, cause diarrhoea or constipation, induce abdominal pain, bloating and distension, and may even be associated with backache, breathlessness, faintness, tiredness, muscle pain, headaches and many other symptoms. Most people with the symptoms of a sensitive gut are diagnosed with irritable bowel syndrome (IBS)[3].

What makes the gut sensitive?

Any disease that causes inflammation of your gut will increase its sensitivity to food, in much the same way as sunburn will make your skin sensitive to the shirt you put on. So people with colitis, Crohn's disease, coeliac disease and diverticular disease can all have symptoms of a sensitive gut when their disease is active, as can people with acute gastroenteritis or food poisoning. Doctors are trained to detect the signs of tissue damage, such as fever, blood loss, anaemia, fatigue and weight loss, but these are not usually present in people diagnosed with IBS. To put it into perspective, coeliac disease is found in only 1% of the British population and inflammatory bowel disease (Crohn's disease and colitis) in less than 0.5%, whereas IBS occurs in 15%.

In the majority of patients, no single disease has been identified to account for a sensitive gut or to explain IBS. Instead, sensitivity may represent a new steady state, a resetting of the brain–gut axis, that may have been caused by a crisis, either a crisis in the gut such as gastroenteritis, or a crisis in a person's life.

For example, an attack of gastroenteritis disrupts the colonic microbiome, alters the permeability of the gut and excites activity in the immune system. These changes affect the production and release of transmitters that act via the gut–brain axis to influence how we feel, not only in our gut but in the rest of our body and mind.

Similarly, depletion of the colonic microbiome by repeat prescriptions of antibiotics may expose the cells lining the gut to harmful, resistant bacteria and activate the gut immune system, causing inflammation and heightened sensitivity. (Microbial depletion may explain why probiotics seem to help a proportion of people with IBS.)

The same cycle of changes can also be initiated by emotion and life events. Stress, trauma, anger, fear, desperation and grief do not only activate the emotional centres of the brain stem, they also stimulate adjacent areas which regulate bodily functions[4], such as eating, digestion, how quickly food travels through the gut and defaecation. All of these can change the composition of gut microflora, which in turn may affect the reactivity of the gut immune system and the information that is relayed back to the brain. Emotional arousal also acts on the brain and the spinal cord to make us more aware of incoming signals from the gut, so even moderate contractions or distension may be felt as pain or discomfort.

GUT FEELINGS; GUT REACTIONS

Emotions are often associated with bodily symptoms, many of which have been adopted as metaphors for the way we 'feel'. Just think of some of the words and phrases we use to describe emotion: 'choked-up', 'fed-up', 'you make me sick', 'I can't swallow that'. It is not by chance that so many of these terms are related to the gut. Emotion is so often expressed as gut reactions. We even use the term 'gut feelings' to describe intuition, and 'gut reactions' for impulsive actions.

Throughout our lives, we all acquire new gut associations. The brain learns by making and breaking connections: nerve cells reach out, connect, break and reconnect. When something happens in association with a gut illness, the brain 'remembers' that connection so that anything that rekindles the memory of that event brings back the symptoms. This may in part explain why IBS sometimes seems to be triggered by a gut infection or life events.

POST-INFECTIOUS IBS

About 10% of people develop persistent abdominal discomfort and bowel upset that can last for years after a bout of gastroenteritis. The infection may have gone, but the memory lingers on in the gut. Gastroenteritis is the most common risk factor for IBS; people who fall ill with gastroenteritis are seven times more likely to develop IBS.

In May 2000, highly dangerous *E. coli* seeped from a farm into a reservoir supplying water to the small town of Walkerton in Ontario, Canada. Over the next few weeks, 1,286 people had severe gastroenteritis with bloody diarrhoea. Over one-third of these suffered persistent gut upset for several years[5]. Analysis showed that

those most affected were more likely to be women with more severe infection and more anxiety and depression during the outbreak.

Biopsies taken from the colons of people with post-infectious IBS have revealed evidence of a persistent mild inflammation, which may be related to a sensitisation of the gut immune system caused by changes in the composition of the microflora (bacteria, fungi and viruses) in the gut, but there is another possibility. There could be no doubt that what happened in Walkerton constituted a major trauma in that quiet rural community, so much so that the trauma etched the gut illness on the brain, so that anything that reminded those affected of what happened rekindled the symptoms of the original infection.

POST-TRAUMATIC IBS

Many people describe how their gut symptoms seemed to be initiated by a particularly upsetting life event[6].

These days, psychologists call the illness that follows an episode of trauma post-traumatic stress disorder (PTSD). After a time, many gain respite from the trauma by blocking it from conscious thought and going into a state of selective amnesia or denial. But the memory does not go away, it hides like a terrorist, primed to effect a campaign of sabotage on the body whenever rekindled by association. Reactions may be experienced as bodily symptoms, without any obvious medical explanation, but with an emotional connection to the original trauma. For victims of PTSD, it is no longer the memory that persecutes their every living moment, their own physiology becomes the source of torment and fear! They are afraid of going to bed, because they wake up tense and sweating, with heart palpitations.

They avoid going out because of the fear of incontinence. They cannot sit down to a meal because everything upsets them. Time does not necessarily resolve the illness. The symptoms are 'the bodily trace left by the trajectory of trauma'[7].

There can be few of us who escape trauma. It may be losing a job, having a serious argument, being involved in an accident or being disappointed in love. Well-meaning friends may advise you to let it go and move on, but our minds do not work like that. Every trauma leaves its imprint, altering the connections between your prefrontal cortex and the emotional centres of your brain, impressing itself on your body as symptoms that represent what happened.

What upsets a sensitive gut?

Whether your illness is initiated by an attack of gastroenteritis, or a particularly gut-wrenching event, what remains is a gut that is sensitive to anything that stimulates it. This may be the food that you eat, or any change or upset in your life.

Food

If your gut is sensitive, any foods that stimulate it will cause symptoms. These include irritants, such as alcohol, hot spices and the hard edges of bran flakes; foods that trigger intestinal spasms such as fats or coffee; poorly absorbed carbohydrates (FODMAPs) in milk, bread and many fruits and vegetables that generate gas or retain fluid in the gut and; or high-fibre foods that add bulk to the colon.

FODMAPS

People have known for a long time that prunes, plums, beetroots and apples cause 'the runs', while onions, artichokes, sprouts and beans are 'gassy'. More than half a pint of milk a day can also cause diarrhoea and wind in those who have lost their lactase enzyme after weaning. But it was not until 2006 that gastroenterologist Peter Gibson and his team at Monash University in Melbourne, Australia, proposed that the poorly absorbed small-molecular-weight sugars in a variety of foods could cause bloating, flatulence, abdominal pain and diarrhoea in people with sensitive guts. For these, they coined the term FODMAPs, an acronym that stands for Fermentable Oligosaccharides, Disaccharides, Monosaccharides and Polyols[1].

As Gibson explained[8], 'FODMAPs are sugars that are poorly absorbed in the small bowel. They drag more water into the gut and are fermented by the abundant bacteria in the large bowel, generating odourless gases (hydrogen, carbon dioxide and methane). The sum effect of these actions is to distend the bowel which, if the gut's nervous system is sensitively tuned (as in people with IBS), may cause bloating, pain and change in bowel habits.' Hence, FODMAPs might trigger symptoms of IBS and reduction of their intake in the diet might then reduce those symptoms.

Whether FODMAPs produce gas or retain fluid depends on their quantities and molecular size, the rate at which they arrive in the colon and the time they stay there, as well as the composition of the microbiome. Smaller sugars, such as the disaccharide lactose, the monosaccharide fructose, and the polyols found in many fruits, tend to retain more fluid in the gut and be voided as diarrhoea, whereas the larger fructo- and galacto-oligosaccharides – found in many vegetables and legumes – are more associated with flatulence and bloating, and only tend to cause loose motions if the colonic microflora is depleted, or excessive amounts are delivered to the colon.

Not everybody reacts to high-FODMAP foods. People who do not have sensitive guts can usually enjoy the whole gamut of fruits, veg, breads and cereals with impunity. And even those with IBS can tolerate many FODMAPs according to their own susceptibilies and the fluctuating sensitivies of their guts.

FODMAPs include the following sugars or groups of sugars:

• FRUCTOSE is present in large amounts in honey and in many fruits. It exists together with glucose, which may stimulate its absorption, but when the amount of fructose exceeds that of glucose, the excess enters the colon. Some may be fermented, releasing gas, while the remainder retains fluid and may be evacuated as diarrhoea.

• LACTOSE is milk sugar. It is a disaccharide, composed of glucose and galactose. In people who lose their lactase enzyme after weaning and have a sensitive gut, undigested lactose may cause discomfort, gas and diarrhoea.

• FRUCTO-OLIGOSACCHARIDES (FOS) are short-chain complex sugars containing strings of fructose molecules. They cannot be digested in the small intestine but are fermented by colonic bacteria, causing bloating, pain and flatulence in people with a sensitive gut. Onions and garlic contain up to 20% FOS. Wheat contains only between 1 and 4% FOS, but this may be significant when wheat is eaten as a staple food.

• GALACTO-OLIGOSACCHARIDES (GOS) are similar to FOS but contain strings of galactose molecules. Most beans and lentils contain substantial concentrations.

• POLYOLS are sugar alcohols (e.g. sorbitol, mannitol, xylitol, maltitol, isomalt). They can be found naturally in fruits including apricots, apples and pears, and in vegetables such as mushrooms, butternut squash and sweet potatoes, and are often added to processed foods. Confectionery contains the highest concentrations. Foods that contain large concentrations of polyols can cause diarrhoea in people with a sensitive gut.

FATS
Fats are one of the most reactive ingredients in the gut. They delay the emptying of the stomach, stimulate contraction of the gall bladder, induce secretion from the pancreas and trigger colonic contractions. People with a sensitive gut are often sensitive to rich sauces, fried food, red meat and creamy desserts, which may cause nausea, bloating, abdominal pain and diarrhoea.

DIETARY FIBRE

Not so long ago, nutritional scientists blamed a highly refined, fibre-depleted diet for IBS, and prescribed a high-fibre diet. Then a series of papers by Dr Peter Whorwell from Manchester University demonstrated that fibre might make symptoms of IBS worse[9], so more doctors now advise a low-fibre diet.

Dietary fibre is a generic term, subdivided into:
- INSOLUBLE FIBRE includes the hard, woody seed coats (such as wheat husks), the cellulose structure of stems and leaves and the skins of some fruits and vegetables. These can be partially digested by colonic bacteria, but the remaining 'roughage' may irritate a sensitive gut and cause pain and loose motions[9].
- SOLUBLE FIBRE includes the beta glucans of oats, pectins, food gums, many beans and vegetables and certain bulk laxatives such as ispaghula as well as a range of resistant starches. They can be fermented by the microbiome, but their large molecular size and viscosity limits the rate of gas production. RESISTANT STARCHES occur naturally in some beans, green peas, rolled oats, pearl barley and unripe bananas. They cannot be digested in the small intestine, but are fermented by bacteria in the colon. They also include wheat, rice and potato starches that have been cooked, cooled and reheated. This tangles and clumps the starch molecules, rendering them resistant to digestion. Since fermentation of these large compacted molecules proceeds relatively slowly, bloating may not be so great a problem as with FODMAPs.

COFFEE

Coffee stimulates the gastro-colonic response, triggering cramping and bowel evacuation in people with a sensitive gut. Tea may have a similar effect in some people.

CHILLI

Chilli directly irritates the sensitive gut, causing cramping and diarrhoea. Most other culinary spices are calming.

ALCOHOL

Consumption of alcohol encourages the growth of harmful bacteria, such as *E.coli*, which break it down to acetaldehyde. This makes the gut more leaky, allowing the toxins that these bacteria produce to invade the gut wall, causing inflammation not only in the gut but throughout the body. Reports suggest that people with IBS can be very sensitive to alcohol. For some, even one drink is enough to cause symptoms for days.

GLUTEN

Many people with IBS find that wheat upsets them and may put themselves on a gluten-free diet. There is no need to go on a strict gluten-free diet unless you have been diagnosed with coeliac disease, but patients with IBS may be sensitive to the fructo-oligosaccharides in wheat[10] as well as to the irritant effect of gluten, so restricting wheat may well help.

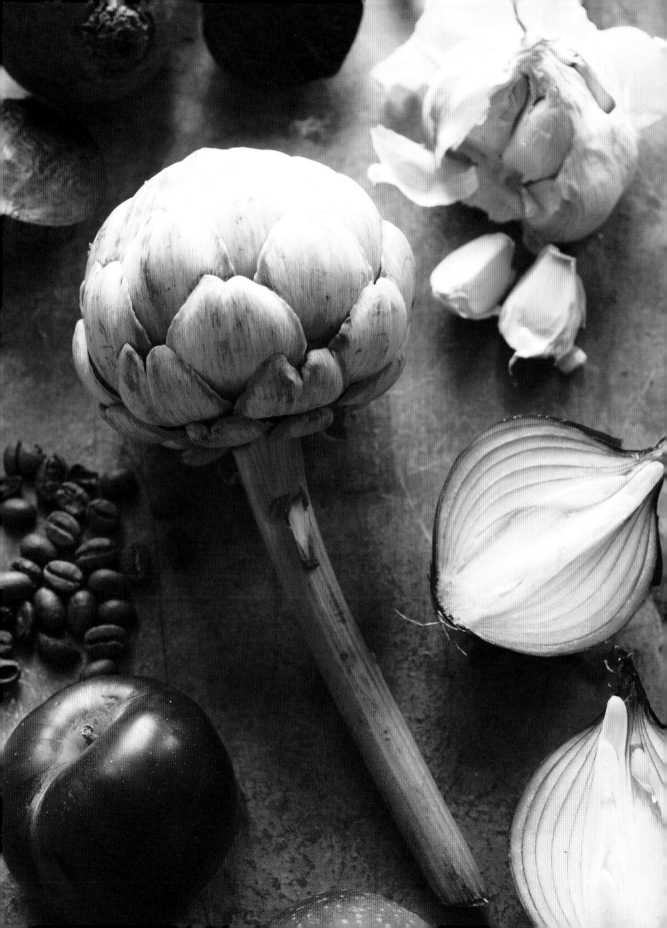

Emotions

Charles Darwin didn't only write *The Origin of Species* and the definitive treatise on barnacles, he also wrote a major monograph entitled *The Expression of Emotion in Man and Animals*, in which he described how the emotions could excite the gut[11].

'When the mind is strongly excited, it instantly affects the state of the viscera, making them blanch with fear or get engorged with anger or excitement, inducing a state of paralysis or stimulating peristalsis and evacuation, or just making them exquisitely sensitive.'

So anxiety, panic, shock, frustration, anger, rage, torment, grief, despair or just working too hard trying to keep it all together can stimulate the sympathetic nerves that go to the gut, causing spasm, pain, bloating, nausea, and bowel upset if your gut is already sensitive.

FACEBOOK, TWITTER AND LIFE ON THE MOVE

Life for many of us these days is conducted at the touch of a screen. Tasks that used to take up much of our time – banking, shopping, meetings – can now be done remotely and much more quickly. This should give us more time to relax, but it doesn't. Now that everything can be done so much more rapidly, we may have the time to devote to many more things, but all of these diverse roles demand our attention, removing time we might otherwise use to focus and think.

Persistent emotional tension makes us all very sensitive not only to what is happening in the outside world, but also to what is happening on the inside. Women are said to pride themselves on their ability to multi-task, answering the phone with an infant in their arms, a toddler screaming in the next room, dinner in the microwave and another email pinging through on the computer, but surely all of this comes at an enormous cost in emotional tension. Does all this tension explain why illnesses of sensitivity such as IBS are so much more common in women?

OTHER PEOPLE

Life affects us, but of the factors that wrench our guts out of kilter, the most common is other people. A cross face, a harsh tone of voice, an aggressive attitude, difficult behaviour, feeling ignored and disregarded… these nuances can all be expressed by your gut feelings and gut reactions. And if the way somebody behaves reminds you of a previous trauma, then it's often your gut that remembers.

Even doctors, the people who should be able to help, can end up making things worse. When tests are negative, drugs fail and reassurance just irritates, patients can all too easily feel a fraud, unworthy of help. If the illness that tortures you every day cannot be validated, what does it say about you as a person?

LONELINESS

In our so-called civilised Western societies, more people are living alone than ever. About 35% of British people now live by themselves with just Facebook or a mobile phone for company. Loneliness is a major cause of illness in our society. Without anybody to talk to, threats or worries can assume enormous significance, especially if the threat is compounded by pain in your gut.

Food and mood

Any change in emotional tension can make the gut more or less sensitive to foods that stimulate it. This explains why food intolerance can come and go according to how you are feeling. Most people with IBS have an erratic pattern of symptoms and bowel habit. Sometimes they are all right; other times their symptoms really play up. Some find they can eat a lot more when they are relaxed on holiday. Others may find that a holiday upsets their gut.

Food is second only to sex in the meaning it conveys. Many vegetarians associate red meat with blood and violence. Chocolate is often called 'naughty'. There is something about shellfish that some associate with sexual intimacy. Chocolate eclairs may carry a burden of guilt, but muesli can seem a puritanical control food. It's often not just what we eat that affects our sensitive gut, but what it represents.

And we are continually assaulted by food scares: red meat contaminated with antibiotics and hormones; vegetables and fruit impregnated with herbicides; fish carrying unacceptable quantities of heavy metals. We are told that the food we eat could harm us and our children. And the more we know, the more anxious we become. So could it be your fear about food rather than any biological action that is triggering your IBS as a self-fulfilling prophecy?

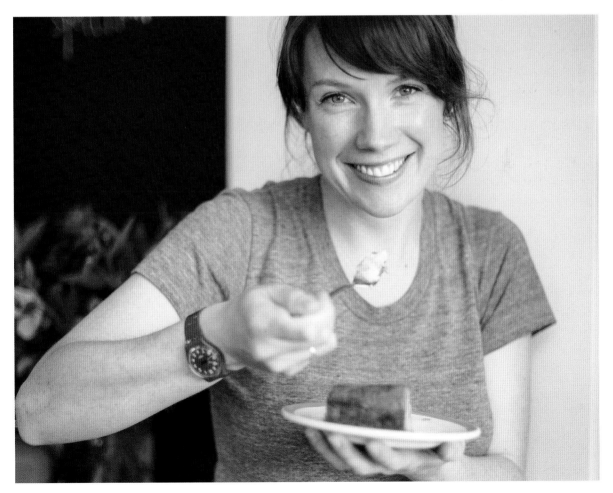

Managing your sensitive gut

There is rarely a quick fix for a sensitive gut. It takes time and patience to rectify a state of excitation in the gut that may have been present for years. You can't go back and undo what has happened. But that doesn't mean it's hopeless. Change is possible, situations improve, memories fade, but in the meantime you can still learn to manage your sensitive gut by medication, stress reduction and, of course, the food you eat.

One of my patients would arrive for every appointment with the same triumphant smile on his face, the same intake of breath through pursed lips and the same sad shake of his head: 'You know the pills you gave me last time? No good! They made me worse!' We were in a therapeutic dance of failure that would only end when one of us walked off the floor. People do best with the symptoms of a sensitive gut when they feel motivated and engaged to do it themselves, with just a few options and a little guidance.

So you need to learn to be your own doctor. After all, you know yourself much better than any health professional can.

SYMPTOM DIARY

To help yourself, keep a diary of what is associated with a flare-up of your symptoms; not only what you eat, but also what occurs in your life. Try to identify your triggers, but also record how any medication, change in diet or other interventions affect your symptoms. How you create your symptom diary is up to you, but we would suggest the following.

First, allow at least two weeks to settle into a pattern of careful cooking and eating based on the recipes in this book, and find space in your day to relax and reflect on what is happening in your life and how you feel about it. Then start your diary.

Log any flare-ups of your symptoms and, alongside, note any changes in what you have been eating or any life events (including whether you have been worrying).

After a time, you should be able to see a pattern emerging. This will inform you what you need to do to rectify it.

You diary will also serve as a baseline to allow you to introduce more foods into your diet and monitor the response of your symptoms.

Lay your symptom diary out something like this:

DATE	SYMPTOM FLARE-UP	CHANGE IN FOOD INTAKE	LIFE EVENT
06.04	Diarrhoea and pain	Half bottle of wine	Argument with Tom
10.04	Pain		Very busy at work
12.04	Bloating and wind	Out for a meal	Late night

MINDFULNESS AND STRESS REDUCTION

When you are stricken with that dreadful combination of physical and emotional symptoms, you are in a vicious spiral: the more anxious or frustrated you become, the worse your symptoms get… and this makes your anxiety worse. Your alarm systems are hyper-aroused, pushed beyond their limits of tolerance. Everything upsets you, even the food you eat. Brain imaging techniques have shown that at those times, the emotional centres in the brain stem are hyperactive and the regulatory systems of the body go haywire, but conversely, the part of the brain that is self aware and keeps the body under control (the medial prefrontal cortex), goes off-line. Emotions and body regulation are out of control.

So remove yourself from the situation. Try to find time and space for yourself. Relax, breathe deeply, close your eyes, silence the tumult in your mind and let the symptoms in your gut subside. And as you relax, be mindful; be aware of how certain thoughts can upset your gut and how your gut symptoms make you feel emotionally.

Mindfulness meditation[12] brings your thinking brain back online, makes you more aware of your feelings and what they mean, and allows you to relax and focus. Body-based therapies, such as yoga or therapeutic massage, can all assist mindfulness, balancing and calming the autonomic nervous system and helping you gain control over your emotional and physical symptoms.

But being mindful does not have to mean sitting in a darkened room and meditating to the sound of gentle music and the aroma of joss sticks. You can be mindful about anything you do: working, reading, walking in the country, playing with the children and – most importantly – cooking. Make these part of your routine and you will feel better.

Food intolerance need not be a life sentence. Just as there will be stressful times when the gut is very sensitive and you will need to watch what you eat, so there will also be times when you feel more confident and you can extend your range. Know yourself, be mindful of what is happening and, with luck and practice, you may find that without you noticing, your symptoms could disappear. It just needs a change in pace and attitude and time to think and practice.

And if there is something that's happened that you cannot come to terms with, or some ongoing situation that is tying your guts in knots, don't struggle on by yourself. Phone a friend. Talk to your husband or wife, your sister, your mother. Just connect to somebody you trust. They will help to get things in perspective. That feeling of being held in mind, feeling connected, understood and cared for is so helpful in calming your symptoms. And if you can't bear to tell somebody you know, make an appointment to see a counsellor or psychotherapist for professional advice and insight.

Eating for a sensitive gut

If you have a sensitive gut, you might think that most of what you eat could upset you. Fortunately, for the vast majority of people with IBS, that is not the case. First, you do not need to eliminate any food, you just need to restrict those that are most likely to cause you problems. Second, the foods that irritate or distend the gut are quite predictable. So it is quite possible to enjoy a varied and nutritious diet while restricting the most irritating or gassy foods. Apart from milk – which most people in

Northern Europe can drink with impunity – these are largely fats, fruits, vegetables and cereals, and also alcohol.

Nevertheless, we are constantly encouraged to eat our five fruits and vegetables a day, to have plenty of fibre in our diet, in order to nourish the good bugs in our guts. Most of the fruits, vegetables and cereals we eat are incompletely digested in the small intestine, and the indigestible residues are fermented in the colon, providing energy and nutrients for our microbiome. This process is very important for our general health. We know that people who eat lots of meat are more at risk of cancer and heart attacks, while a highly refined diet containing few fruits or vegetables may lead to obesity or diabetes.

So the very foods that are so good for our general health can aggravate a sensitive gut. The gas generated and the fluid retained by poorly absorbed sugars (FODMAPs) may make the symptoms of pain, bloating and diarrhoea worse. If you have IBS, you just can't win… or so it seems. But Peter Gibson and his team from Monash University, in Melbourne, Australia, have a solution: the low-FODMAP diet.

THE LOW-FODMAP DIET

The principle of the low-FODMAP diet for IBS is to restrict the fruits, vegetables and cereals that are rapidly fermented and produce so much gas, while maintaining an adequate intake of dietary fibre that is more slowly fermented, feeds the bacteria and keeps the bowels moving. The low-FODMAP diet works, at least in the short term, probably because it restricts all possible sources of rapidly fermented carbohydrate. Trials have shown that eliminating or restricting FODMAPs reduces bloating, abdominal pain and diarrhoea in about 70% of people with IBS[1]. This might

be a placebo effect, but the fact that symptoms returned when patients were challenged with FODMAPs sugars without their knowledge, suggests that it wasn't.

We might wonder whether such a restrictive diet is necessary. After all, most people from Northern Europe can absorb lactose; fructose absorption may be facilitated by the glucose present in most fruits, honey, and in some high-fructose corn syrups; and the tolerance of fat and responses to fructo-and galacto-oligosaccharides show enormous variation between individuals and within an individual at different times. Feed more fructose and more will be absorbed. It's all about individual susceptibility and tolerance and maintaining a sense of balance. As Peter Gibson commented: 'many do not need the strict diet in the longer term, but can remain well with few symptoms with only some restriction, such as avoiding onions and consuming only small quantities of wheat-flour-based products.'[8]

Going on a restricted diet is potentially hazardous. The danger is that you will eliminate so many foods that your diet will become depleted of energy and essential nutrients. This is a particular risk for vegetarians, or those already on strict 'free-from' diets. That is why dieticians recommend that the elimination phase of the low-FODMAP diet is monitored by a trained dietician and followed by piecemeal reintroduction of each restricted major component. But there are just not enough dieticians to help and monitor everybody who might need it. Moreover, there are few long-term data on the success of reintroduction. We have therefore adopted a different approach. We have demonstrated how easy it is to prepare appetising and healthy meals, using low-FODMAPs ingredients, as a baseline from which you can gain confidence and adapt the recipes to best suit you and your sensitive gut.

Why 'cooking for the sensitive gut'?

The ultimate success of any change in diet depends on the extent to which you can understand and adapt it to suit yourself. Regulation and control rarely work. Make something too difficult, or too compulsory, and people will inevitably find ways to defeat it. In our experience, diets only work if you can learn from them to make a long-term adjustment in lifestyle that makes you feel good. For any change to work, you need to understand it, believe in it, and feel inspired and motivated to persevere with it. It needs to become part of who you are and the way you live. Too many people are passive recipients of a health-care system that has no definite answer to illnesses like IBS, that are an expression of the individual, their life experience and the way they live. You need to take control of your sensitive gut, using your health-care professionals for advice and reassurance where necessary.

It is never easy adjusting your diet to restrict so many familiar foods, especially if the sensitivity of your gut changes with whatever is happening in your life, but neither is it rocket science. Cooking engages you in your own treatment. You are in control. Once you have learned a recipe, you can adjust the ingredients and portion sizes and find what suits you and when.

There are no foods that are strictly off limits for people with a sensitive gut, though there are many that may need to be restricted. Everybody is different, there is enormous variation in the rate at which food moves through the gut, the degree of absorption, the pattern and extent of fermentation, not to mention the emotions certain foods induce. And there is also huge disparity in the foods that we eat, not just the species of plant they are from, but which part of the plant you eat, the strain, the ripeness, the storage and the way it is cooked; they all influence the way the food might affect you. You can't expect any health professional to know what is going to suit you and when. They can only give general guidance as to what kinds of foods might upset you and then leave it up to you.

You know yourself better than any doctor. Cooking for yourself means you can be in control of what you eat, explore your limits of flexibility and try things out. For example, most people living in the UK can tolerate dairy. Moreover most natural sources of fructose also contain roughly equivalent amounts of glucose which may facilitate fructose absorption. This means that, even if you have IBS, you should be able to enjoy an apple, or some honey in your porridge or on a slice of toast. Most fruits contain very small amounts of polyols and even one or two prunes and apricots can be cut up and sprinkled on your porridge. Similarly, one or two cloves of garlic added to a dish should not upset you. You know the science; it's a matter of gaining confidence with a restricted diet and then exploring your own personal range.

The recipes in this book follow current dietary advice for IBS. They limit those foods that contain substantial amounts of FODMAPs, they are low in the fatty foods that may upset a sensitive gut, and they avoid chilli, coarse wheat bran and coffee. They are a safe start, from which you can adapt and expand your range of foods as you gain confidence and experience, so you can gradually come to define your own diet. Our aim is to help you find out what you can eat, not tell you what you can't.

And just because your gut may be sensitive from time to time doesn't mean you can't have a varied, interesting diet. Variety is the hallmark of balanced and healthy eating and, as the recipes in this book show, it is quite possible to enjoy a great number of appetising dishes.

Our recipes are not necessarily the final solution for your sensitive gut. Only you can discover that. But they will put you on a safe track to find the foods that work well to keep you healthy and symptom-free.

So try the ones you like. Learn a few new tips and techniques. Get used to them. And as you become familiar with your favourites and develop confidence, explore your range of flexibility. Under less stressful circumstances, you and your gut have a wide degree of adaptability. Increase the amount of fructose in your diet, or some of the polyol components, and your gut will adapt to absorb more. Increase the intake of fat and your gut will become less sensitive to it.

It is not just the amount of a single 'gut stimulant' in any meal that counts, but the total amount of stimulants in the meal. So some people with IBS may be able to tolerate a small amount of beetroot but if this is eaten in a salad with lentils, beans, avocado and rocket, the total load of fermentable carbohydrate may exceed the gut's capacity to deal with it in comfort. A sensitive gut will not tolerate too much food at once.

And remember, your sensitive gut is very much an interaction between your mood, how you feel, and the food you eat. A happy and confident gut is much less likely to complain.

Although we have done our research, we cannot promise you that none of the recipes featured in this book will upset your gut. We are what we eat... and what we don't eat. Our guts are as individual as our brains in the way they respond to their environment. Above all, learning to cook for your sensitive gut is an education, not only about your diet but also about you.

IT'S NOT JUST WHAT YOU COOK, IT'S THE WAY THAT YOU COOK IT

Cooking is the ideal way of developing a comfortable relationship with food. It requires a relaxation and focus, attention to ingredients, process and timing. Setting aside 20 minutes or so to create a meal, savouring what you have prepared with your family, enjoying that sense of togetherness, is an everyday art form; an exercise in mindfulness.

If you can develop a good relationship with food, then this extends to other areas of your life, such as work, responsibilities and other people, especially those closest to you. It is an attitude of a mind that works by association.

So this is more than a recipe book. It uses cooking as mindful metaphor to achieve a greater sense of self-awareness. The recipes are a means to an end: the restoration of health confidence and harmony.

But enough of the theory... It's time we got cooking!

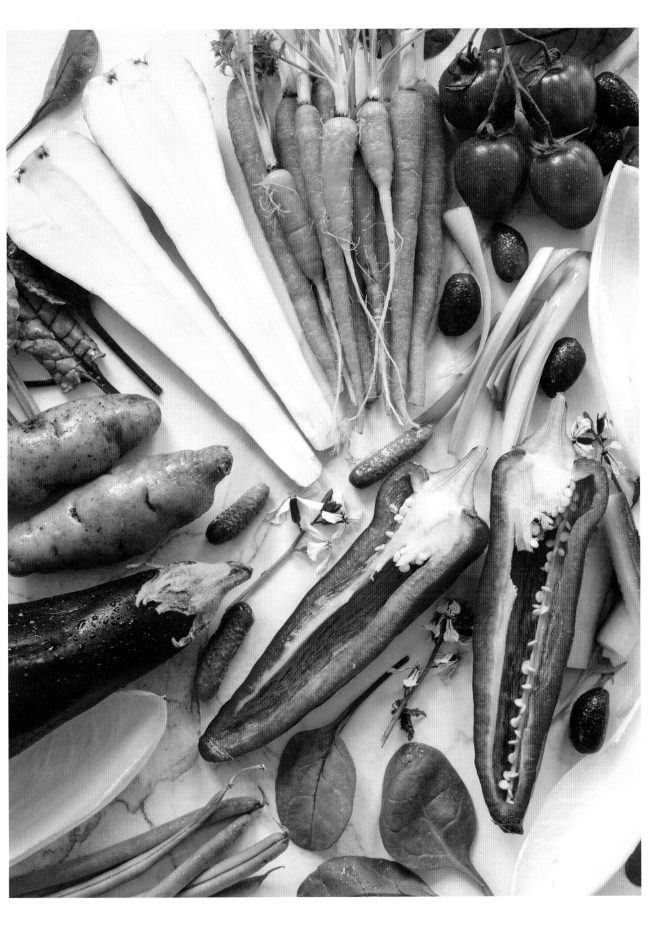

Gut-friendly foods

The good news is that there are many foods you can eat if you have a sensitive gut. The thing they all have in common is they are low in FODMAPs and in fat, coarse wheat bran, chilli and other ingredients that might stimulate or irritate. We have tried to include as great a variety of natural foods as possible, maximising your chance of obtaining all the nutrients you need to remain healthy.

Changing your store cupboard and fridge to include more gut-friendly ingredients will help you manage your symptoms better and make preparing and eating food a real pleasure. Our recipes will also help you to manage your weight and eat a balanced diet that supports your overall health.

We have used a traffic light system to indicate the foods that you can eat in moderate amounts and those that you need to restrict. All foods in the green category can be eaten and used in our recipes in moderate amounts; those in the amber category should be eaten and used in restricted quantities; only very small portions of the foods in the red category should be eaten. For example, you can eat a small slice of regular white bread from the red category (more if you are using spelt sourdough, see page 54). This might not seem much, but it is a useful amount in cooking: it means you can include breadcrumbs in a crisp topping for fish, include a few in meatballs, or indulge in a slice of toast every now and then. Although some of the ingredients in our recipes may stimulate a sensitive gut, we have either restricted the portions to amounts that would not be expected to cause symptoms, or suggested alternatives.

This traffic light system is just a guide. Just because a particular food is in the red zone, it doesn't mean you can't ever eat it, or, indeed, that you can always eat a food in the green zone. The reality is that it depends on the individual. People vary and we want to encourage you to experiment within your own personal boundaries and find out what best suits you.

As you become familiar with some of the recipes, we would encourage you to be more flexible with the portion sizes to find out what works for you.

FISH, MEAT AND EGGS

Fish, lean meat and eggs are important sources of protein and should be included regularly in a gut-friendly diet. Although salmon is known as 'oily fish', its fat content is relatively low. Fatty cuts of meat, sausages, rich stews and sauces that contain high amounts of fat should be avoided or eaten in small portions. Sausages and other processed meats often contain cereals and onions, which can both upset a sensitive gut.

Sausages

Fattier cuts of pork and lamb

Chicken, lean beef, lean lamb, lean pork and lean bacon
Fresh and smoked oily fish, such as salmon and mackerel
White fish, such as cod, haddock and hake
Shellfish such as prawns and crab
Canned fish such as anchovies, salmon and tuna
Chicken's and quail's eggs

CEREALS AND FLOURS

Cereals are an important source of energy and you should include a serving in each meal.

Wheat, barley and rye contain low concentrations (1–4%) of fructo-oligosaccharides (FOS). Thus small amounts may be tolerated by most people with a sensitive gut: a small portion of pasta, one slice of toast, or wheat flour used as a thickener for a sauce. Other cereals, such as rice, maize, buckwheat and quinoa, contain lower amounts of FODMAPs and so more can be tolerated. We have included spelt sourdough bread because it contains much lower concentrations of FOS, so more can be eaten. We occasionally use gluten-free flour because it is often made from a mix of flours other than wheat (rice, potato and maize), which contain lower amounts of FOS.

Regular white bread, rye bread, wheat flour, barley flour

100% spelt bread, pasta, oats

Buckwheat flour, cornflour, gluten-free flour, maize flour, oat bran, polenta, potato flour, rice flour

Gluten-free pasta, rice (white, brown, red or wild), quinoa

Rice cakes, oat cakes, tortilla chips (plain)

Gluten-free bread, 100% spelt sourdough bread

100% buckwheat noodles, rice noodles, glass (mung bean) noodles

MILK, YOGURT, BUTTER AND CREAM

80% of people of Northern European background living in the UK retain the enzyme that breaks down lactose and can tolerate milk and yogurts even if they have a sensitive gut, though the fat in whole milk products may give problems. But people of Asian, Southern European or Afro-Caribbean ethnicity are more likely to be lactase-deficient as adults and may be intolerant of lactose if they have a sensitive gut. Most people who are lactase-deficient still produce a small amount of the lactase enzyme. Tolerance varies and small amounts of milk may be added to tea or coffee, but larger amounts may be problematic.

Lactose-free cow's milk and plant milks made from soya, rice and oat may be used instead of regular cow's milk. Cream contains a minimal amount of lactose and a small portion can be tolerated by most people intolerant of lactose. Whole milk, butter and calcium are rich in fat, which may upset people with a sensitive gut. Coconut milk is much lower in fat than cream and is a good alternative to cream in soups.

In live yogurts, milk sugar is partially fermented and the amount of lactose reduces with the length of storage. Two tablespoons of regular plain yogurt can usually be tolerated by people who are lactose intolerant.

Milk, yogurt and cheese are important sources of calcium and should be included regularly in the diet. You do not need to restrict your intake of milk if you know you can absorb lactose. If you do malabsorb lactose you might consider taking liquid drops, tablets or capsules with lactase substitutes which can reduce your symptoms by helping your body break down any lactose in your diet more easily. Lactase substitutes can either be added to milk or taken just before eating a meal. They can be obtained from chemists and health food shops.

Buttermilk

Cow's milk, whipped cream, sour cream, yogurt, butter

Lactose-free yogurt, lactose-free milk, soy milk, oat milk, almond milk, coconut milk

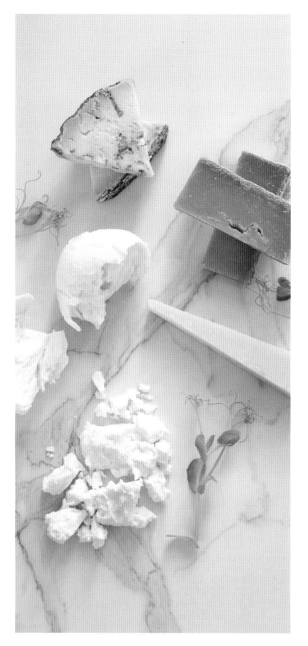

CHEESE

Small portions (20–30g/1 oz) of hard cheese are fine for most people since they contain little lactose. All the great cooking cheeses such as Cheddar, feta, goat's cheese, mozzarella and Emmental are suitable for our gut-friendly recipes. However, a third of the weight of most cheese is fat, which may trigger symptoms if too much is eaten.

Softer, younger cheeses such as ricotta and cream cheese do contain some lactose, but can be eaten in small portions.

Cream cheese, ricotta, halloumi

Camembert, Cheddar, cottage, Emmental, feta, goat's, Gruyère, mozzarella, Stilton and other blue cheese

HERBS AND SPICES

Chilli

Black pepper, fennel seeds

Spices including asafoetida, cinnamon, coriander seeds, five spice, root ginger, liquorice, nutmeg, star anise, turmeric

Herbs including angelica leaves, basil, chervil, chives, coriander, dill, elderflower, lemon verbena, mint, parsley, rosemary, sage, sweet cicely, tarragon, wild garlic

FRUIT

Fruit is our major source of vitamin C and contains important amounts of dietary fibre. It is therefore essential for a healthy diet and at least two portions should be eaten every day. But fruits are also a rich source of FODMAPs (fructose, polyols and fructo-oligosaccharides). The FODMAP content of fruit varies according to the type of fruit, the variety, how it has been stored and how ripe it is.

It is best to eat just one piece of fruit at a sitting (approximately 80 g/3 oz). You can enjoy a mix of fruit throughout the day but, to be safe, allow time to digest one piece of fruit before eating another. Drying fruit concentrates the fructans and fructose in fruit, so it is best to limit your intake of dried fruit to 1 tbsp of raisins or sultanas.

Apples, apricots, avocados, blackberries, cherries, figs, grapefruits, mangos, nectarines, peaches, pears, persimmons, plums and prunes

Currants, raisins, sultanas, desiccated coconut

Bananas (ripe, but not overripe), blueberries, cranberries, grapes, kiwi fruits, lemons, limes, cantaloupe and honeydew melons, oranges, papayas, passion fruits, pineapples, raspberries, rhubarb, strawberries

VEGETABLES AND PULSES

Vegetables are an important source of vitamins, minerals and dietary fibre. At least three portions a day are advised for a healthy diet. Although several contain significant amounts of fructo- and galacto-oligosaccharides, there are many that can be eaten by most people with a sensitive gut.

Pulses are an important source of protein for vegetarians and vegans, but most are high in fructo- and galacto-oligosaccharides. There are exceptions. Canned lentils and chickpeas contain smaller amounts and can be eaten by most people in modest portions, such as 2 tbsp. It is important to rinse canned pulses well before using them in recipes as this washes off any fructo- and galacto-oligosaccharides that have leached into the canning water. 1 tbsp of green or red lentils, cooked at home, should also be tolerated by most people.

Artichokes (Jerusalem), asparagus, beetroots, cauliflowers, garlic, mushrooms, onions, peas, shallots, the white part of salad onions and leeks, all pulses (apart from those listed below)

Artichoke hearts (canned), broccoli, butternut squashes, celery, chickpeas (canned), lentils (canned and home cooked), sweet potatoes

Aubergines, capers, carrots, celeriacs, chard, chicory leaves, courgettes, cucumbers, endives, fennel bulbs, ginger, green beans, kale, leeks (green leaves only), lettuces, olives (black and green), pak choi, parsnips, peppers (red, orange, green), potatoes, radicchio, rocket, spinach, spring onions (green leaves only), swedes, tomatoes, turnips, water chestnuts, watercress

NUTS AND SEEDS

Nuts and seeds are nutritious ingredients that contain protein, fat and many vitamins and minerals. They are also a useful source of dietary fibre. Most can be eaten in small portions (about 1 tablespoon) without causing symptoms. Linseed and chia have a gelatinous coat that swells up when soaked in water and these seeds are a gentle way of stimulating the bowel if you tend to be constipated.

Cashews, pistachios

Almonds, fennel seeds, hazelnuts

Chia seeds, linseeds, macadamias, peanuts, pecans, pine nuts, pumpkin seeds, sesame seeds, sunflower seeds, walnuts

Almond butter, peanut butter

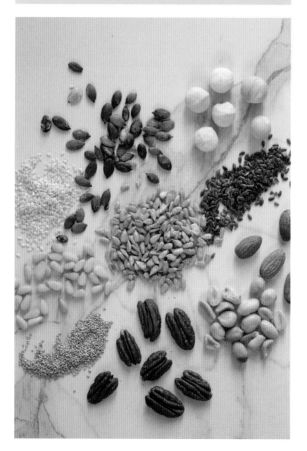

SWEETENERS

Sugar (sucrose) and glucose are easily absorbed in the small intestine and are well tolerated, although for general health these sugars should be limited in the diet. Honey contains a lot of fructose, which is slowly absorbed if it occurs in excess of glucose, and may cause symptoms such as abdominal pain and loose motions if too much is eaten. However, in most honeys, the proportion of glucose to fructose is roughly equivalent so more could be tolerated. Artificial sweeteners sometimes contain sorbitol and xylitol which are also poorly absorbed and should be avoided if present in large amounts. Sugar-free chewing gum often contains high concentrations of sorbitol. Check food labels for these ingredients.

Fructose, honey, agave nectar, artificial sweeteners ending with 'ol' such as sorbitol, mannitol, xylitol

Golden syrup

Glucose, maple syrup, sugar (white, brown, caster, icing)

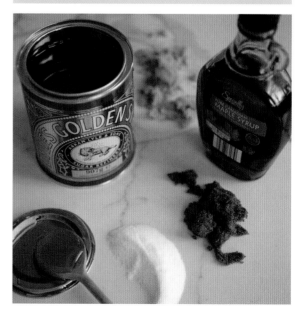

BASICS

Getting prepared

Make sure you have a good set of kitchen appliances. This will make your life so much easier. We cannot do without the following:

- Digital kitchen scales so that you can get to grips with portion sizes.
- Measuring jugs for liquids.
- Timer so that you time cooking and get the best results.
- Immersion/stick blender to make smoothies and soups.
- Juicer to make fresh fruit and vegetable juice.
- Food processor to help you chop, mix and purée ingredients.
- Electric hand mixer for making cakes.
- Spiralizer or julienne cutter to make vegetable spaghetti.
- Grater for grating cheese, lemon and orange zest.
- Good-quality potato peeler.
- Large pestle and mortar for grinding spices.
- A set of good-quality non-stick pans including a large frying pan with a lid. Non-stick pans make cooking with the minimum amount of fat possible while retaining the flavour of the food. Reducing the amount of fat in your diet is very important if you have a sensitive gut.
- Steamer – great for cooking vegetables such as spinach, kale, young carrots and potatoes.
- Wok for stir-frying.
- A large pot for making stock and cooking pasta.
- Knives: a 20cm/8 in chef's knife, a small, 10cm/4 in vegetable paring knife.
- Tongs.

A few tips before you start

- Preparing food from scratch is easier if you get organised. Arrange the store cupboard so that the ingredients you use frequently are most accessible. Keep your kitchen appliances within easy reach.
- Read a new recipe all the way through before you start. This will fix it in your mind, so you know what you are doing and can get organised and work quickly.
- Follow the recipe closely the first time you make a dish. Then, when you cook it again, you can alter the portions and ingredients to suit you. The recipe then becomes yours.
- Weigh all your ingredients. You will not only get better results, but all of our recipes have been formulated to contain the amounts that you can tolerate without feeling ill.
- In preparing a meal, timing is everything. Plan it out beforehand. While the main component of your meal is in the oven, you can be chopping and steaming vegetables, making a sauce, preparing a salad. Be mindful, focus, relax and enjoy.
- Use your timer. While bread is proving, you can be doing something else and the timer can remind you when it is time to attend to the dough for the next stage. Timers on phones and tablets are great because they are portable and can be taken round the house with you.

Onions and garlic

So many dishes rely on onions, but white and red onions, shallots, garlic and the white part of leeks and spring onions (scallions) all contain high amounts of fructo-oligosaccharides (FOS). If you suffer from IBS, it is important to restrict their use, but with a little ingenuity it is possible to get that flavour without upsetting the gut.

The green leaves of leeks and spring onions can be used in place of the white parts, or of whole onions. As the plant grows, the green leaves break down the fructans present in the bulbs of onions, leeks and garlic. (Baby leeks include comparatively more green leaves and are a less wasteful way of using leeks.)

We also recommend growing and using chives and garlic chives. They have a delicate fresh flavour and you can chop off their long, thin blades and add as many as you need to a recipe to get the right taste for you. They are easy to grow even in a window box.

Some cooks use asafoetida to pep up dishes cooked without onions, but many do not like its pungent, bitter flavour. Asafoetida is used very sparingly in Asian cooking and it may be worth a try if you have a robust palate.

The fructans in garlic may be tolerated better because they are not fermented so easily. If you like the flavour of garlic, one or two cloves in a recipe can often be fine for IBS sufferers. And, since garlic has such a strong flavour, less may be needed. For salads, try rubbing a garlic clove around the salad bowl to flavour the ingredients as you toss them.

The leaves of wild garlic are an ideal alternative to garlic cloves. They have a more delicate flavour and should not trigger symptoms.

Another option is to use garlic-infused oil which can be bought or made at home. (It has a short shelf life so needs to be used quickly.)

Garlic-infused oil

The FOS in garlic are soluble in water, whereas the allicin and other volatile compounds that give garlic its distinctive aroma are soluble in oil. Thus the gorgeous, aromatic flavour of garlic can be extracted by steeping sliced garlic in oil and then straining it out before using.

You can make garlic oil as and when you need it. Either fry a couple of cloves of sliced garlic in enough olive oil for a recipe, then discard the garlic and use the flavoured oil within a day.

Or just slice two cloves of garlic and leave them covered with olive oil for an hour. Strain out the garlic and use the oil within a day. (The same method works if you want to infuse vegetable oil instead, which is more authentic in Asian dishes.)

Both methods capture the wonderful flavour of garlic, but each oil tastes slightly different. The raw garlic-infused oil is nice in salad dressings, while the cooked version is better suited to add to tomato sauce in pasta dishes.

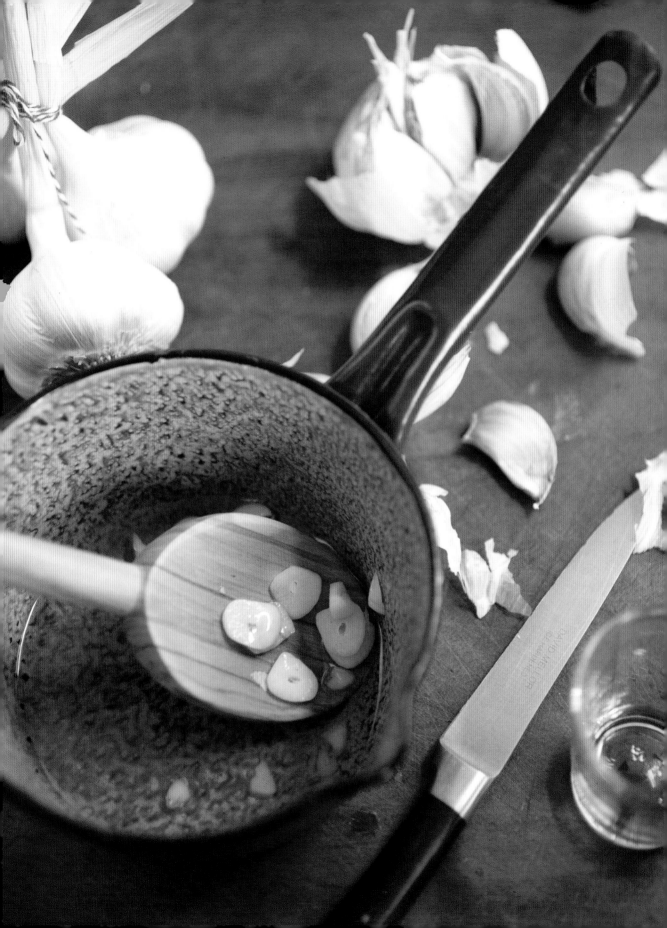

Polenta two ways

Polenta is made from maize flour (cornmeal) and is a staple food in northern Italy. It is a great substitute for pasta in Italian meals that contain the strong flavours of basil, red (bell) peppers or tomatoes. It is tolerated by most people with a sensitive gut because maize is gluten-free and low in FODMAPs.

Quick-cook polenta takes about 10 minutes and can be served 'wet' or 'firm'. Wet polenta is cooked to the consistency of porridge and can be enriched with a little butter or cheese. It is served with casseroles and sauces, or topped with vegetables. Firm polenta is cooked to the consistency of mashed potato, then tipped out of the pan and allowed to cool and set. It is then cut into pieces and either brushed with oil and fried, or grilled, so it develops a delicious crisp crust but remains soft inside. This polenta can be served chopped up as croutons with soups and salads, or eaten as a snack sprinkled with Parmesan cheese and fresh herbs.

SERVES 6 FOR A MEAL (with leftovers to grill or bake)
Hands-on time 10 minutes
Cooking time 10 minutes, plus 2 hours to set firm

sea salt and freshly ground black pepper
225 g/8 oz/1½ cups quick-cook polenta
50 g/2 oz/½ stick unsalted butter
50 g/2 oz/½ cup Parmesan cheese, finely grated, plus more to serve
a little olive oil, for the tray and to cook (if making firm polenta)

Bring water to the boil in a pan, according to the polenta packet instructions, salt the water well, then gradually whisk in the polenta. As soon as the polenta starts to boil, it 'blips' like a volcano, so place a lid on the pan. Reduce the heat and simmer the polenta for about 10 minutes or according to the packet instructions. The cooked polenta should have the consistency of porridge.

For wet polenta, remove it from the heat at this stage and stir in the butter and Parmesan. The wet polenta is now ready to serve with a final sprinkle of Parmesan. If you are particularly sensitive to fat, you could just serve the wet polenta with small dots of butter and a sprinkle of Parmesan cheese rather than stirring butter and cheese into it.

For firm polenta, continue to cook until it reaches the consistency of mashed potato. Spoon the polenta on to a lightly oiled baking tray and, using a palette knife, spread it into a rectangle about 2.5 cm/1 in thick. Leave to set for at least 2 hours. Cut into wedges, brush with a little olive oil and grill, or fry in a non-stick pan. Any extra can be wrapped in cling film (plastic wrap) and stored in the fridge.

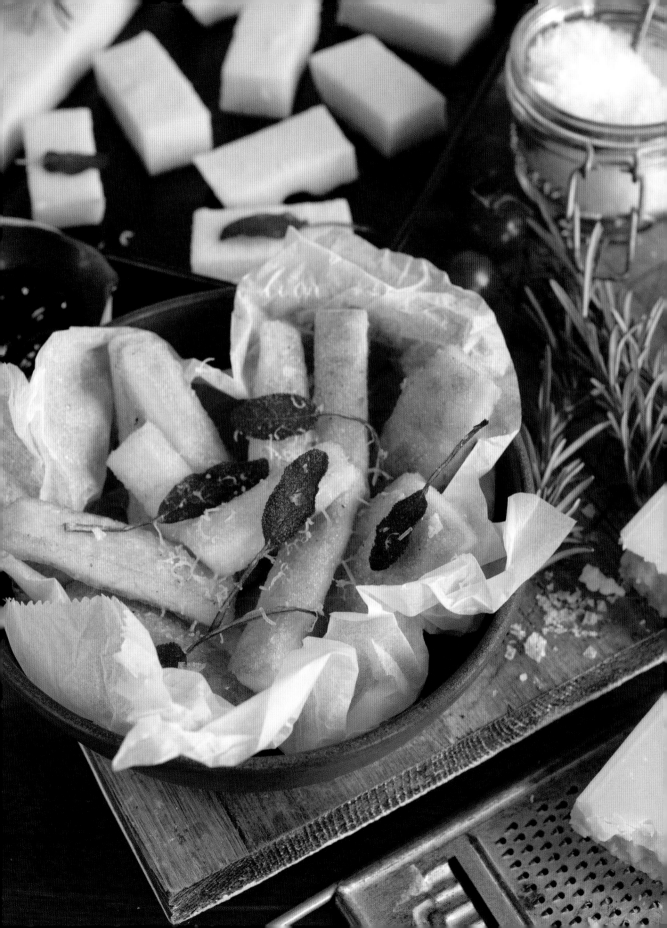

Pasta

75 g/3 oz/½ cup of cooked pasta (about half a regular portion) is low in FOS and should not trigger symptoms in most people with a sensitive gut. You can always make it up to the equivalent of a full portion of pasta by supplementing with one of the following options.

If you are gluten-sensitive and feel more confident cutting wheat from your diet, one option would be to substitute polenta for pasta (see p.38). This works really well with Italian dishes that include a sauce, such as Bolognese. Or you could do a straight swap with gluten- and wheat-free pasta, though we have not yet found a version we like; we prefer buckwheat or rice noodles.

Or why not think outside the box and make 'pasta' from potatoes, or courgettes? A spiriliser gadget can cut long spaghetti-like strands of vegetable 'pasta' (see p.82). Spiralised potato and courgette make 'pasta' you could eat with Bolognese or tomato sauces, while spiralised carrot, cucumber and courgette make salads. This is a really fun option!

Rice

Rice can be eaten by anybody with a sensitive gut. It does not contain gluten and is low in FOS. Some may find the more fibrous brown rice causes symptoms and, if it does, stick to white rice. Short-grain rice can be used in puddings. Arborio and carnaroli rices are excellent in risottos, while basmati is perfect for stir-fries and South-East Asian dishes.

We love using different kinds of rice and one of our favourites is black rice, available in health stores and online. It releases a nutty aroma as it cooks and is pleasantly chewy. We also love red Carmargue rice and wild rice. These all take longer to cook than white rice; we use at least three times the volume of water to rice and allow 25 minutes.

The recipe below is the perfect way to cook wonderfully fluffy basmati rice using the absorption method.

SERVES 4
Hands-on time 1 minute
Cooking time 12 minutes

175 g/6 oz/1 cup basmati rice
½ tsp salt

Place the rice in a small saucepan with twice its volume of water and the salt. Bring to the boil, cover with a tight-fitting lid, and leave to simmer on a very low heat for exactly 12 minutes. Do not be tempted to take the lid off, as the rice is happily cooking in the steam created under the lid. Uncover after 12 minutes; there should be no water left, but you should be able to see little steam holes. Lift a few grains with a fork and taste them to see if they are cooked. Return the lid to the saucepan and leave the rice to steam off the heat for a couple more minutes, then fluff up the grains of rice with a fork and serve.

ALTERNATIVE METHOD
Wait for the rice to boil, cover and let it steam, undisturbed, in the covered pan for 20 minutes.

Making good stock

A good stock is the basis of a well-made soup or stew. We always recommend you make your own stock from bones, vegetables and herbs. Not only is the flavour so much richer, but you can be more confident of the ingredients. For example, you can use the green leaves of leeks and spring onions, or chives or wild garlic, as a substitute for onions.

Home-made stock needs at least an hour of gentle cooking in a large saucepan for the flavours to develop. If you have any leftover stock, you can reduce the volume by simmering on the hob. It can then be cooled and frozen in ice-cube trays or plastic cartons. Stock will last for two months in the freezer.

However, if time is short, you can also try using organic stock powder or granules and keeping it quite dilute. Most stock powders do contain onions, though, so see how you get on.

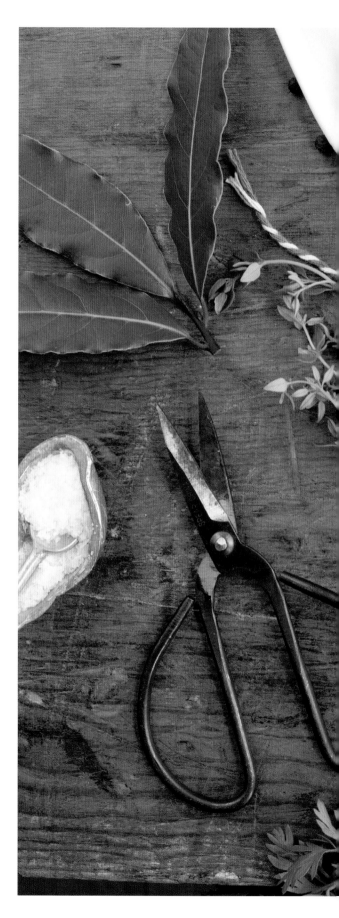

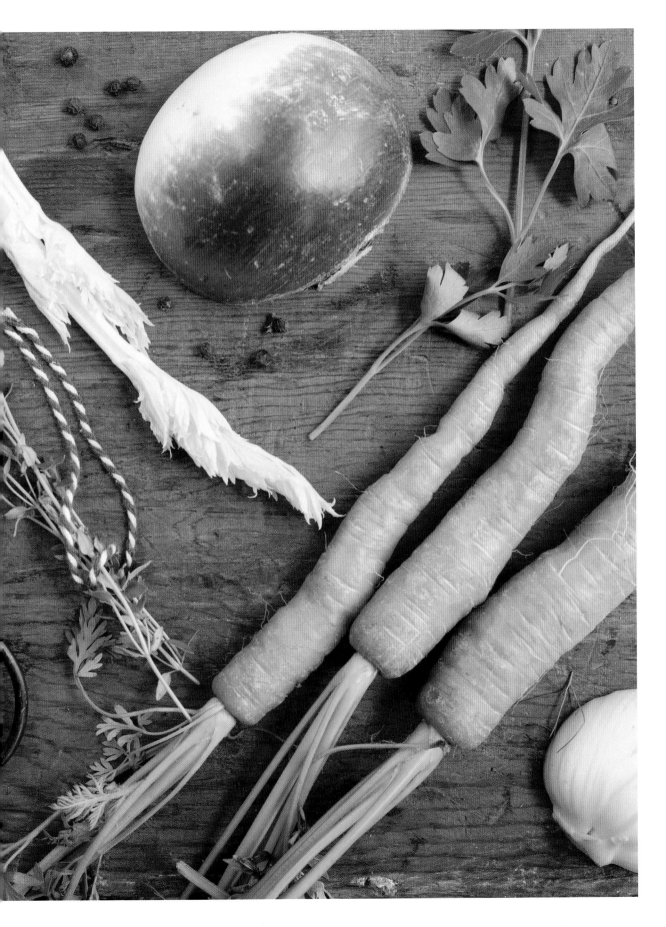

Our basic stock

We love this vegetarian stock. It has a gentle fragrance and forms the basis of all the delicious soups in this book. The blend of herbs gives it a lot of flavour. This recipe contains thyme, parsley and bay leaves, but other herbs such as tarragon would be lovely both here and in the chicken or fish versions that follow.

MAKES 2.5 L/4.5 PINTS/
2.5 QUARTS
Hands-on time 15 minutes
Cooking time 1 hour

green leaves from 3 young leeks
4 large carrots, peeled
1 fennel bulb, or its discarded
    stalks and fronds
2 celery stalks
1 small turnip
2.5 litres/4.5 pints/2.5 quarts of
    cold water
small bunch of parsley
2 bay leaves
small bunch of thyme
10 black peppercorns

Wash and roughly chop all the vegetables and place in a large, deep saucepan with the water.

Add the herbs and peppercorns and bring to the boil. Reduce the heat and allow to simmer gently for 1 hour.

Remove from the heat and allow to cool. You can strain and use the stock at this point but, if you have time, cool the stock, place in the fridge and allow the vegetables to continue to infuse for a further few hours, then strain and use. Remember to cool and freeze any extra stock.

FOR CHICKEN STOCK
Add the bones from a chicken carcass. The stock will need to be simmered for about 1½ hours, then drained. It should look clear and be an amber colour. Cool the stock before storing it in the fridge for up to 4 days, or freezing in ice cubes or small plastic containers for up to 2 months.

FOR FISH STOCK
Add 1 kg/2 lb 4 oz (at least 4–5 medium carcasses) of broken-up white fish heads and bones, such as plaice or haddock. The stock will need to be simmered for 15 minutes, without letting it boil, or it will turn cloudy. Cool and strain the stock before storing it in the fridge for up to 4 days or freezing in ice cubes or small plastic containers for up to 2 months.

White sauce

A smooth, velvety white sauce is the basis of some really fine dishes such as fish pie, lasagne or fillings for stuffed pancakes. A classic white sauce starts with equal quantities of flour and butter cooked gently together, then let down with cow's milk, though lactose-free or plant milks can be used instead.

The amount of wheat in a white sauce should not trigger symptoms in most people, but, if you want to try to make a wheat-free white sauce, rice flour or cornflour (cornstarch) are good substitutes. Rice flour gives a slightly rougher texture, but we like it because it doesn't form lumps. With cornflour you have to keep stirring to keep lumps at bay.

If you have time, you can infuse herbs and other aromatics into the warm milk; if you don't, the sauce will still be good but with slightly less flavour.

MAKES 570 ML/1 PINT/
2⅓ CUPS
Hands-on time 10 minutes
Cooking time 10 minutes,
    plus 30 minutes to steep the
    herbs in milk (optional)

FOR THE SAUCE
570 ml/1 pint/2⅓ cups lactose-
    free milk
30 g/1 oz/2 tbsp unsalted butter
30 g/1 oz/¼ cup rice flour,
    cornflour (cornstarch)
    or plain flour
sea salt and freshly ground
    black pepper

TO FLAVOUR THE MILK
    (OPTIONAL)
2 bay leaves
½ celery stalk, roughly chopped
1 tsp black peppercorns
1 tbsp chives, roughly chopped

If you want to flavour the milk, place the milk, bay leaves, celery, peppercorns and chives in a saucepan and bring to the boil. Remove from the heat and allow the herbs and aromatics to infuse in the warm milk for 30 minutes. Strain the milk.

Gently melt the butter in a saucepan. Add the flour and stir until the mixture forms a thick paste (known as a roux) that leaves the sides of the pan. This should take about 2 minutes. Gradually add the milk, a little at a time, stirring continuously. Continue to stir and cook the sauce until it thickens and coats the back of a spoon. Season to taste.

Basic tomato sauce

The mainstay of Italian cooking and many delicious Middle Eastern dishes. It is a really useful sauce and worth making carefully.

We love home-made tomato sauce with big, bold, herby flavours such as rosemary, bay, oregano and basil. To make up for the lack of onion, we have packed this sauce with other great complementary flavours such as anchovies, which just melt into the background, a little dry white wine, capers and olives. This sauce is lovely with our Courgetti (see p.82) or with buckwheat noodles.

SERVES 4
Hands-on time 15 minutes
Cooking time 30 minutes

2 tbsp olive oil
1 garlic clove, sliced
½ celery stalk, finely chopped
1 small carrot, peeled and
    finely grated
400 g/14 oz can of plum
    tomatoes
2 bay leaves
sea salt and freshly ground
    black pepper
a few torn basil leaves

OPTIONAL INGREDIENTS (ADD
    IN ANY COMBINATION)
4 anchovy fillets in oil
1 glass (150 ml/5 fl oz/⅔ cup) dry
    white wine
1 tbsp capers, drained and rinsed
1 tbsp olives, roughly chopped

Warm the olive oil in a saucepan and add the garlic. Cook until the garlic begins to brown, then remove it from the pan and discard. Add the celery and carrot. If you are using anchovies, add them at this point and allow them to melt into the sauce. Or you can add the wine and allow it to evaporate.

Add the plum tomatoes to the saucepan and break them up with a wooden spoon. Swill the empty tomato can with a little water and add the water to the sauce.

Drop the bay leaves into the sauce and season well. Capers and olives, if using, can be added at this point.

Cook the sauce gently for at least 15 minutes in a covered pan and then for a further 5 minutes without a lid. This allows it to thicken to the required consistency. Taste and serve with the basil.

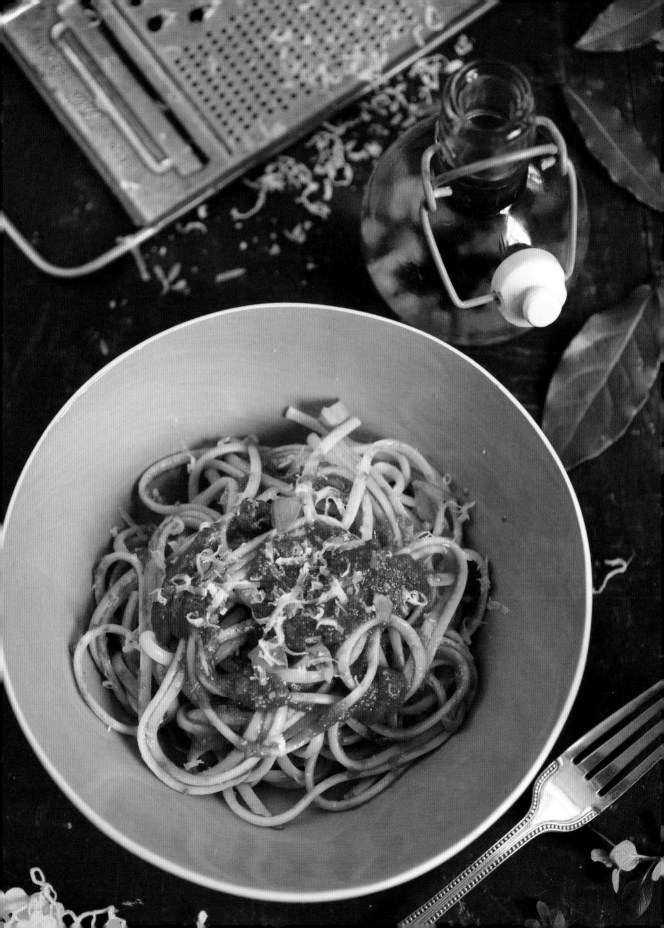

Pesto

Pesto is the heady, cheesy, nutty sauce from Genoa in northern Italy with the peppery perfume of fresh-picked basil. It is the best sauce for pasta, Courgetti (see p.82) and any roasted, warm-climate vegetables such as aubergines (eggplants) and peppers. It is also delicious drizzled over a bowl of soup. Pesto bought in jars has been pasteurised, which can make it taste sour. It is much better to make it fresh.

The Italian word 'pesto' means 'pounded' and recipes for it vary. It does not have to be too garlicky, just a hint will do. You can rub the cut surface of a garlic clove around the dish you are serving the pesto in, or use a little Garlic-infused oil (see p.36). When wild garlic is in season, you can add a few leaves of it with the basil.

This is a really useful sauce and if you feel like no more than a few noodles or pasta for supper, a drizzle of pesto will transform it into something special.

SERVES 4
Hands-on time 5 minutes

50 g/2 oz/½ cup pine nuts
50 g/1½ oz/½ cup Parmesan
   cheese, finely grated
leaves from 1 medium-sized
   bunch of basil
100 ml/3½ fl oz/½ cup olive oil
sea salt and freshly ground
   black pepper

Grind the pine nuts in a mortar and pestle (or food processor), add the Parmesan and about half the basil. Pound these together, then add the remaining basil. Continue to pound these ingredients until they have been broken down to a rough paste.

Gradually stir in the olive oil and season to taste with salt and pepper.

TRY THIS
• *Add the juice and finely grated zest of ½ lemon.*
• *Use Garlic-infused oil (see p.36) instead of olive oil.*

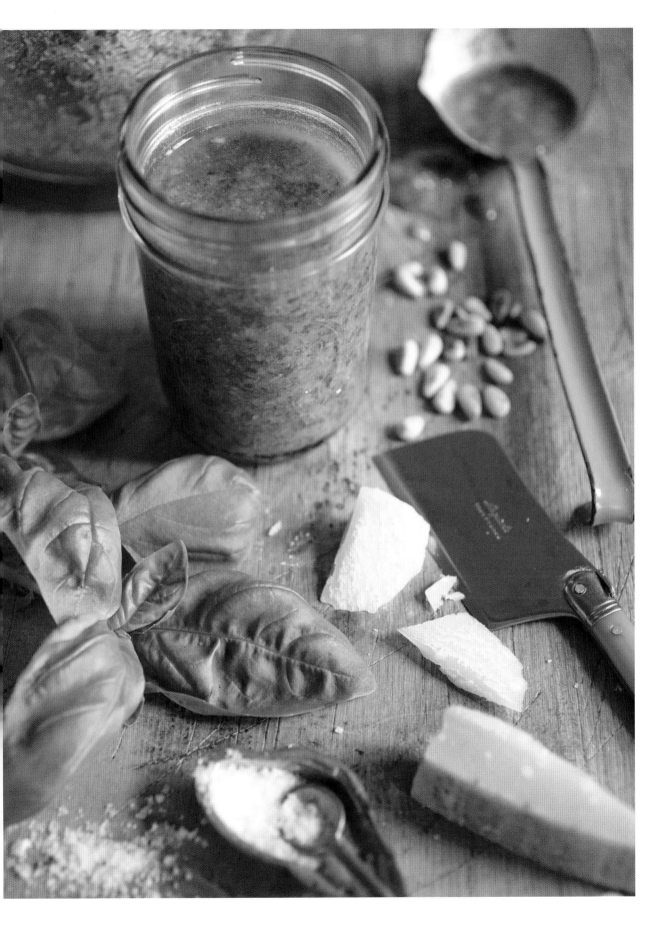

BREAD

Although many people report an intolerance to wheat or a sensitivity to gluten, very few have coeliac disease and so need to follow a strict wheat- or gluten-free diet. (Though to be safe, everybody who finds that bread upsets them should have a blood test for coeliac disease.) Some may indeed have a sensitivity to gluten (though the evidence for such a diagnosis is controversial). Instead, it seems that most people who have symptoms after eating bread are sensitive to the fructo-oligosaccharides (FOS) in wheat. Although wheat flour contains only small amounts of FOS, if large amounts of bread are eaten as a staple food, it may cause symptoms. People with a sensitive gut can usually tolerate a slice of toast or bread at a sitting, or breadcrumbs used to coat fish – and many can cope with more – but if wheat is a problem, there are alternatives.

More than 80% of the bread eaten in the UK is made using the Chorleywood Process, devised in 1961 as a quick way of making bread from flour with a lower protein content. Bread made using the Chorleywood Process takes only three and a half hours to make, compared to at least nine hours using traditional long fermentation techniques. The length of the fermentation time is crucial to the taste and texture of bread and its fructan content. Bread made using the Chorleywood Process tends to have a 'pappy' texture, bland flavour and contains higher amounts of FOS than bread made using traditional slow fermentation methods. The fructans naturally present in flour are used by the yeasts during fermentation. Therefore, certain sourdough breads made from flours such as spelt are low or moderate in fructans. However, sourdough breads made from high FODMAPs flours (such as wheat and rye) are still high in FODMAPs, though anecdotal evidence suggests they are better tolerated by people with a sensitive gut.

Although sourdough rye bread contains FOS, some people may find they can tolerate it better than regular bread. This is thought to be due to the longer chain length of the carbohydrates, which some people find easier to digest. Also smaller quantities of rye sourdough bread are eaten because, although delicious, it is harder to chew and it takes longer to eat.

A good option, if you have time, is to make your own bread, using 100% spelt flour or – even better – make Spelt sourdough bread (see p.54) which is much lower in FOS.

Making bread is all about mastering techniques such as weighing accurately, judging the consistency of dough, learning how to prove a loaf, shaping it, then finally judging when it is baked. If you make bread regularly, it will soon become a satisfying part of your weekly routine and you will be turning out appetising loaves quickly and cheaply. Many people get a huge amount of satisfaction and joy from making bread, but it does take a bit of practice.

If you make several loaves at the same time, they freeze well and can be defrosted when needed. And remember, any leftover bread can be made into breadcrumbs and used in other recipes.

Gluten-free bread

Gluten-free flours can be made from many types of grains and starches such as rice, maize, buckwheat and potato. Not only are they gluten-free, they are also much lower in FOS than regular wheat flour.

Since bread dough made from these flours does not contain gluten, it does not have to be kneaded. Just mix the ingredients together and leave the dough to rise in the loaf tin before baking.

This is quite a forgiving recipe as far as the flour is concerned. If you do not have all of the different flours required, you can adjust the ingredients. As long as you maintain the overall weight of flour and you have at least three of the varieties, the bread will work. This loaf is great eaten fresh and can be toasted the next day when it is not so fresh. It can also be frozen for up to two months.

MAKES 1 LARGE LOAF OR
2 SMALL LOAVES

Hands-on time 15 minutes
Cooking time 30 minutes,
    plus 1½ hours proving time

125 g/4½ oz/1 cup potato flour
125 g/4½ oz/1 cup brown
    rice flour
50 g/2 oz/⅓ cup buckwheat flour
100 g/3½ oz/⅔ cup coarse
    maize flour
1 tsp salt
40 g/1½ oz/¼ cup sunflower
    seeds
40 g/1½ oz/¼ cup pumpkin
    seeds
40 g/1 ½ oz/⅓cup linseed
2 tbsp sesame seeds
2 tbsp poppy seeds
1 tsp fast-action dried yeast
400 ml/14 fl oz/1⅔ cups
    lukewarm water
flavourless vegetable oil,
    for the tin or tins

In one bowl, mix the flours, salt, seeds and yeast together. Pour in the water and mix with a wooden spoon. The mixture will be quite wet and sticky. There is no need to knead the dough. Cover and rest it for an hour in a warm place (21°C/70°F).

By this time, the dough should have risen well. Transfer the mixture to the oiled loaf tin or tins, cover with a clean plastic bag or cling film (plastic wrap), and leave to rise for 30 minutes. It should rise 1–2 cm/½–1 in during this time.

Preheat the oven to 240°C/475°F/gas 9. Place a cup of water in a roasting tin at the bottom of the oven (this helps bread to rise).

Place the bread in the oven, immediately reduce the temperature to 220°C/425°/gas 7 and bake for about 30 minutes. The loaf should be golden brown and, when turned out of the tin, the base should make a hollow sound when tapped. If the loaf is not cooked, return it to the oven for a further 5 minutes. Turn out on to a cooling rack and leave to cool.

Overnight white

This is a simple spelt loaf, made overnight. Spelt is an ancient grain with a nutty flavour and produces excellent bread. Records show it was cultivated in the Middle East 12,000 years ago and, by Roman times, had become popular throughout Europe.

Spelt bread is less likely to trigger symptoms in a sensitive gut than regular bread made from wheat, because it has a lower FOS content, especially if you allow a longer proving time to break down the fructans. Spelt can be bought as wholemeal or white flour and either can be used to make the loaf below. Spelt does contain gluten, so it is not suitable for anyone with coeliac disease.

This dough is quick to mix up and needs only a small amount of attention, but does require time to rise. Start making the bread the night before you want to eat it, leave it to rise overnight, then bake it the following morning.

We love this loaf for its beautiful open texture, wonderful nutty flavour and great toasting and keeping qualities.

MAKES 1 SMALL LOAF
(FILLS A 450 G/1 LB LOAF TIN)
Hands-on time 15 minutes
Cooking time 35 minutes,
    plus 10 hours proving time

300 g/11 oz/2⅓ cups white or
    wholegrain spelt flour, plus
    more to dust
¼ tsp fast-action yeast
1 tsp salt
200 g/7 fl oz/¾ cup lukewarm
    water
vegetable oil, for the tin
2 tbsp seeds, such as pumpkin,
    sesame, poppy, flax (optional)

The evening before you want to eat the bread, place the flour, yeast and salt in a bowl and mix together. Gradually stir the water into the flour with a wooden spoon, then use your hands to bring the mixture together to form a ball of dough.

Cover the bowl with cling film (plastic wrap), or a clean plastic bag, and leave for 10 minutes. Now it is ready to knead. Spelt flour is one of the easiest flours to knead as it develops its elasticity quickly. Keeping the dough in the bowl, pull a portion of it up from the side, then press it back it into the middle of the dough. Spelt dough is quite stretchy so this should be easy. Turn the bowl slightly and repeat the process with another portion of dough. Repeat about 8 times, or until you have worked around all the dough. This should take about 10 seconds.

Cover the bowl again and let it rest for 10 minutes. Repeat this kneading and resting process twice.

Give the dough a final knead (you have kneaded it 4 times in all), cover and leave to rise overnight in a cool (15°–18°C/59°F–64°F) place so that it doesn't over-prove. The dough should have doubled in volume by the morning.

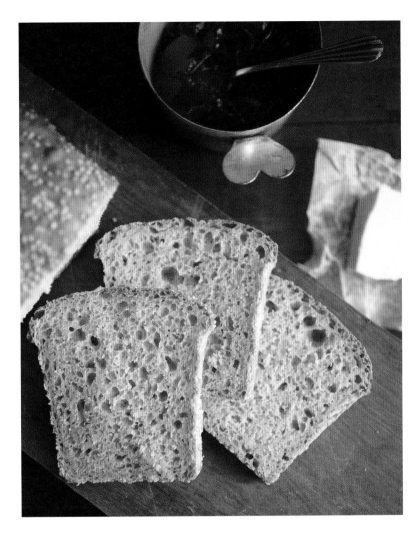

The next morning, uncover the dough and, while it is still in the bowl, punch it with your fist to deflate the dough ball.

Lightly dust a work surface with spelt flour. Remove the dough from the bowl and place it on the floured work surface. Gently pull into an oval shape and fold both ends over into the middle. You will now have a rectangular shape. Pull and fold the top of the rectangle one-third of the way towards the middle, turn round 180° and keep folding until you have a shape the size of a 450 g/1 lb loaf tin. Oil the tin with vegetable oil.

Sprinkle the seeds, if using, on the bread at this point.

Place the dough in the prepared loaf tin, cover with cling film, or a plastic bag, and leave in a warm place to rise to almost twice its original size (about 45 minutes).

About 15 minutes before the bread has finished rising, preheat the oven to 240°C/475°F/gas 9, or as high as it will go. Place a roasting tin at the bottom of the oven filled with a cup full of water. When the oven is up to temperature, remove the loaf's plastic covering and place it in the oven, immediately reducing the temperature to 220°C/425°F/gas 7. Bake for about 35 minutes or until the surface is nicely browned. Turn the loaf out of the tin, tap on the base to check it sounds hollow (this shows it is cooked) and place on a wire rack to cool.

Once you have mastered the simple kneading process above, you can go on to make your own sourdough spelt bread.

Spelt sourdough bread: making the starter

Sourdough bread contains only three ingredients: flour, salt and water. To make the bread rise, you need to create a starter from the natural yeasts and bacteria present in the flour and the air.

The natural yeasts and lactobacilli, along with the long proving time, break down the FOS in the dough so that fewer are available to be fermented in your body.

It will take five days to make the starter and it will keep indefinitely, provided you look after it. We find it performs better the older it is.

Stage 1:
making the sourdough ferment

Day 1. Mix 1 tsp spelt flour and 2 tsp water in a clean jam jar. Seal and leave overnight in a warm place.

Days 2, 3, 4 and 5. Add 1 tsp spelt flour and 2 tsp water to the jar and stir. Gradually bubbles will start to appear on the surface of the mixture. Leave a little longer if the ferment does not look very frothy. This ferment is ready to use when large bubbles appear on the surface.

Stage 2:
making the sourdough starter

Mix 15 g/1 tbsp of the bubbling ferment from stage 1 with 150 g/5 oz/1¼ cups spelt flour and 150 g/5 fl oz/⅔ cup lukewarm water in a large bowl. Leave to ferment overnight. The next day use this starter for your recipe.

Keeping your sourdough

Add 1 tsp of spelt flour to the jar containing the remaining sourdough ferment. Stir well, seal and refrigerate for another time. Putting the ferment in the fridge does not kill the wild yeasts, but causes them to become dormant (sleepy). When you are ready to use the sourdough again, pour away any grey liquid that may have formed and continue to make up the starter as described in stage 2. A fresh influx of water and flour will invigorate the wild yeasts and they will be ready to use again in your next batch of bread.

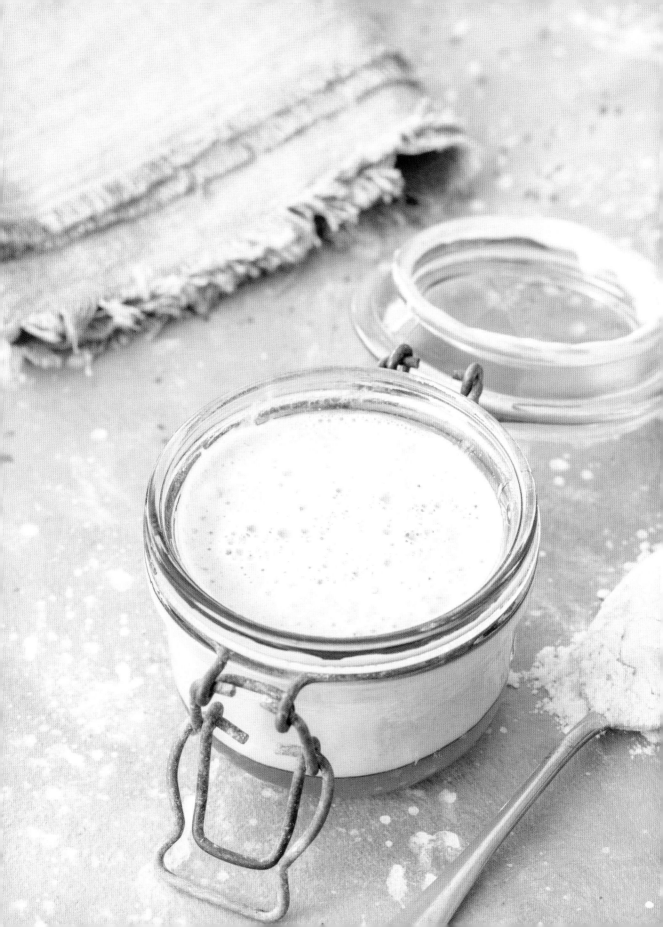

Spelt sourdough bread: making the bread

The only tricky part of making this bread is adding the correct amount of water to the dough. This depends on the type and age of the flour, so you might have to add a little more or less to get the consistency just right. The dough should be stretchy, smooth and a little bit sticky. It is important to slash the top of the loaf before it goes in the oven, to allow the steam generated from within the loaf to push the crust upwards and give the baked loaf a good height. One really useful tip, from a master baker, is to place the dough in the fridge for about 30 minutes after it has risen and before it is baked. This helps the loaf to keep its shape after turning out of the proving basket and makes it easier to slash the top just before it goes in the oven.

MAKES 1 SMALL LOAF

Hands-on time 10 minutes

Cooking time 35 minutes,
    plus 1 day proving time

250 g/9 oz/2 cups white spelt
    flour, plus more to dust
4 g/½ tsp salt
100–125 ml/3½–4 fl oz/⅓ –½ cup
    lukewarm water
75 g/3 oz/⅓ cup sourdough
    starter (see p.54)
a little flavourless oil, for the tray

You will need a 500 g/1 lb
    proving/dough-rising basket
    or a colander and a clean linen
    tea towel

Place the flour and salt in a bowl and mix together. In another bowl, place 100 ml/3½ fl oz/⅓ cup of the water and the starter and mix well. Add the liquid to the flour and mix well. If it is too dry, add some of the extra water until the dough comes together into a soft ball. Use your hands to help at this stage. Cover the bowl with cling film (plastic wrap), or a clean plastic bag, and leave for 10 minutes.

Knead the sourdough (see p.52) and leave the dough to rise for an hour, or until it has doubled in size and feels springy to touch.

Lightly dust a work surface with flour. Remove the dough from the bowl, place on the work surface and shape into a smooth round disc. Line a proving basket or colander with a clean linen tea towel. Dust generously with flour and lay the dough inside. Sprinkle the top of the dough with flour. Allow the dough to rise until it has almost doubled in size. This will take 3–6 hours, depending on the temperature of the air. When the dough has finished rising, place it in the fridge for about 30 minutes. This helps the loaf to keep its shape.

About 15 minutes before baking, preheat the oven to 240°C/475°F/gas 9. Place a roasting tin at the bottom of the oven filled with a cup of water.

Tip the dough out of the proving basket on to a lightly oiled baking tray. Snip a circle around the top of the loaf with scissors, or simply slash it with a very sharp knife. Place the loaf in the preheated oven, then immediately reduce the oven temperature to 220°C/425°F/gas 7. Bake the loaf for about 35 minutes or until the surface is nicely browned. Turn the loaf out of the tin and place on a wire rack to cool.

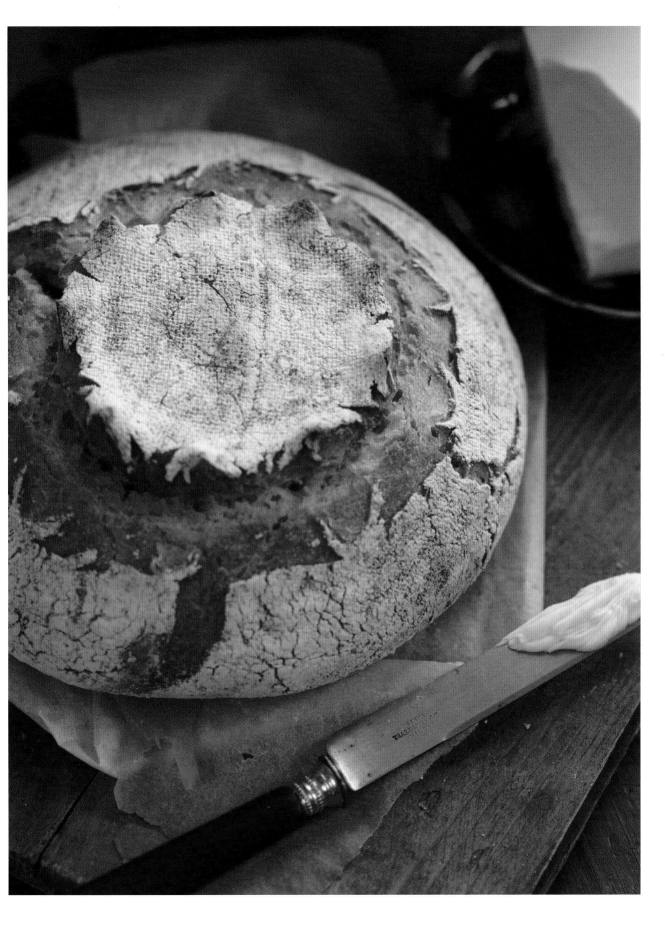

BREAKFAST

A good nourishing breakfast sets us up for the day, replenishing carbohydrate stores that have been depleted overnight. There is evidence to show that a good breakfast helps people focus and work more efficiently.

But what to eat for breakfast can be a difficult choice if you have a sensitive gut. Most commercial breakfast cereals are high in fructo-oligosaccharides (FOS) and many also contain wheat bran that may irritate the gut wall. Milk may also cause symptoms in people who are intolerant to lactose.

But there are alternatives. Breakfast does not have to be based on wheat products. It can include small amounts of oats, rice, quinoa or maize, which, with the texture and taste of seeds such as chia, sunflower, pumpkin and linseed, can provide a satisfying meal that is also good for your gut. And if you cannot tolerate cow's milk, there is always lactose-free milk and a wonderful range of tasty plant milks. Our favourite is almond milk.

Many people enjoy a slice or two of toast for breakfast. This may not be a problem for your sensitive gut, but, if it is, try bread made from spelt flour or our nutty-tasting Spelt sourdough bread (p.54). You could also try our Gluten-free bread (p.51) which substitutes other flours for wheat flour and is lower in FOS than regular bread.

Preserves such as marmalade are not a problem for sensitive guts; neither are savoury spreads such as yeast or meat extract. Honey contains a high percentage of fructose, but it also contains the glucose that eases fructose absorption. So if you love honey, just a smear on your toast or a teaspoonful in your porridge will probably not bother you; you may even be able to tolerate more.

Although few working people have time to cook breakfast during the week, it is nice to relax over a cooked breakfast at the weekend. But you may need to make some adjustments if you have a sensitive gut. Fried breakfasts can contain a lot of fat. Grill the components instead, or just use a smear of fat in a good-quality non-stick pan. Cut the rind off the bacon, avoid fried bread and watch those sausages: regular sausages contain 25% fat and are padded out with cereals, usually wheat. You can of course make your own lower-fat, cereal-free sausages; we have a good recipe (see p.109). Tomatoes are great, but go easy on the mushrooms, because they contain a sugar alcohol called mannitol that is not well absorbed by the gut and may trigger symptoms.

Low-lactose yogurt

It is easy to find lactose-free milk in supermarkets but less easy to find plain, simple lactose-free yogurt. If you are lactose intolerant, your body should be able to tolerate about 2 tbsp of plain yogurt. This recipe allows you to eat a little more. It is smooth, gentle and a little bit creamy and it can be flavoured with a few drops of vanilla extract or a drizzle of maple syrup. It can also be served with a spoonful or two of strawberry jam stirred through. You will need to use 'live' yogurt as a starter, since this contains the bacteria required for it to set.

MAKES 800 ML/1½ PINTS/
3¼ CUPS
Hands-on time 5 minutes
Cooking time 5 minutes,
    plus up to 8 hours to set

800 ml/1½ pints/3¼ cups whole
    lactose-free milk
3 tbsp plain 'live' (regular cow's
    milk) yogurt

You will need a kitchen
    thermometer and one large or
    two small sterilised jars.

Sterilise one large or two small jars: wash the jar and the lid (removing the rubber seal if there is one) and place in a preheated oven at 130°C/250°F/gas ½ for 20 minutes until dry. Simmer the rubber seal in boiling water for 10 minutes, then remove it with tongs and leave to dry.

Heat the milk gently in a saucepan until it reaches 85°C/185°F on a kitchen thermometer. Remove the saucepan from the heat and allow the milk to cool to 43°C/109°F. This will take about 15 minutes.

Stir the 'live' yogurt into the cooled milk and pour into the prepared jar/jars. Cover the jars and set aside in a warm place such as an airing cupboard for about 8 hours. When the yogurt has set, it can be stored in the fridge for up to a week.

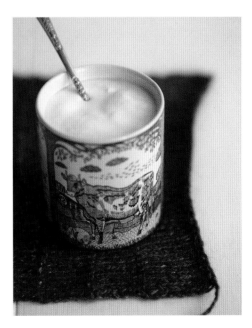

Oat porridge with fruit and toasted seeds

Rolled oats are made from the steamed and rolled kernels (groats) of oats from which the hulls and stalks have been removed. Although they contain some fructo-oligosaccharides (FOS), just a small amount of rolled oats (23 g/¾ oz/¼ cup) can be transformed into a decent bowlful of porridge or muesli. The outer layer of the oat kernel, known as oat bran, is particularly high in a soluble fibre called beta-glucan which retains fluid and gently stimulates a stubborn bowel.

Oats are not only kind to the gut; they have other well-established health benefits such as helping to reduce blood cholesterol.

This simple porridge is the mainstay of many nourishing, familiar breakfast menus. Its viscosity means that it is digested slowly and can be relied on to stave off hunger until lunchtime. The lovely thing about porridge is that you can add other ingredients to vary the taste. Plant milks, such as almond or soya, can be substituted for regular cow's milk. Nuts, seeds and fresh fruit can be added, too.

SERVES 4
Hands-on time 10 minutes
Cooking time 10 minutes

90 g/3 oz/scant 1 cup rolled oats
600 ml/1 pint/2½ cups lactose-
   free milk or water
2 tsp seeds, such as sunflower,
   pumpkin seeds, linseed
100 g/3½ oz chopped fruit,
   such as blueberries,
   strawberries, kiwi fruit,
   raspberries or oranges
1 tsp vanilla sugar (optional)

Place the oats in a saucepan with the milk or water and bring to the boil. Reduce the heat to a simmer. Cook the porridge for 4–5 minutes, stirring continuously, until it reaches a creamy consistency.

Meanwhile, heat the seeds in a frying pan and toast, stirring, until they are just turning brown.

Remove the porridge from the heat and stir in the seeds. Top with chopped fruit and dust with vanilla sugar, if you like.

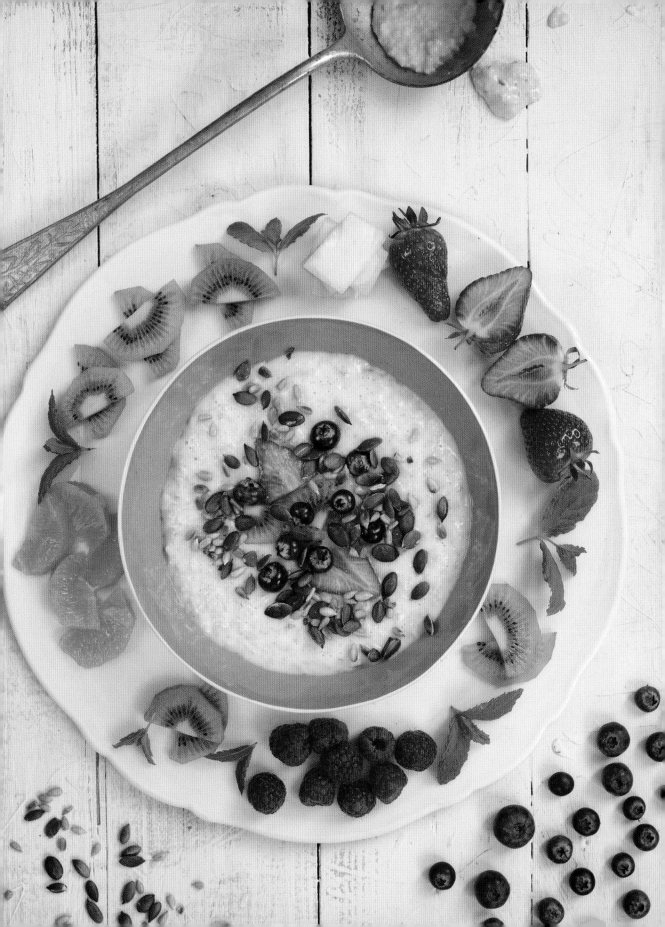

Granola pots

Granola is a wonderfully crunchy mix of seeds and cereals toasted with a coating of syrup. It usually contains dried fruits, but we have reduced these since most contain polyols, fructose and fructo-oligosaccharides (FOS). The only exception is raisins, which can be eaten in small amounts (1 tbsp), so we have sneaked some in. Maple syrup is a delicious way of sweetening this recipe, but can be expensive. Golden syrup is a good substitute and more economical, but it does contain some FOS, so go easy on it. Granola makes a great breakfast, but can also be eaten as a snack, scattered over fruit and yogurt, or added to crumble toppings.

SERVES 6
Hands-on time 15 minutes
Cooking time 15 minutes

FOR THE GRANOLA
150 g/5 oz/1½ cups rolled oats
60 g/2 oz/½ cup almond nibs
    or flakes
60 g/2 oz/½ cup walnuts
60 g/2 oz/½ cup pumpkin seeds
1 tbsp flax seeds
30 g/1 oz/⅓ cup desiccated
    coconut
3 tbsp maple syrup
    or golden syrup
2 tbsp vegetable oil
1 tsp vanilla extract
4 tbsp raisins

FOR THE STRAWBERRY
    COMPOTE
140 g/5 oz/1 cup strawberries,
    hulled and roughly chopped
1 tbsp caster (superfine) sugar,
    or to taste
1 tsp lemon juice, or to taste
yogurt, to serve
chopped fruit to serve, such
    as blueberries, strawberries,
    raspberries or kiwi fruit

Place all the dry ingredients (except the raisins) in a bowl. In another bowl whisk together the syrup, oil and vanilla. Pour the wet ingredients over the dry ingredients and mix, making sure the oats and seeds are well coated.

Preheat the oven to 200°C/400°F/gas 6. Spread the mixture out loosely on a baking tray and bake in the preheated oven for 15 minutes. Halfway through, stir the granola and check it is not scorching around the edges. Continue cooking until it is just turning golden brown; do not be tempted to cook it for too long.

When the granola is removed from the oven it is soft, but it hardens as it cools. Stir the raisins into the granola when it has cooled and store in an airtight container.

For the compote, place the strawberries in a saucepan with the sugar, lemon juice and 1 tbsp of water and cook gently for about 10 minutes. The strawberries should be soft but still retain some shape. Allow to cool a little before tasting, then add a little more sugar or lemon juice if you like.

To assemble the granola pots, place 1 tbsp of strawberry compote in a glass serving dish, followed by a sprinkling of granola. Top with yogurt and chopped fruit.

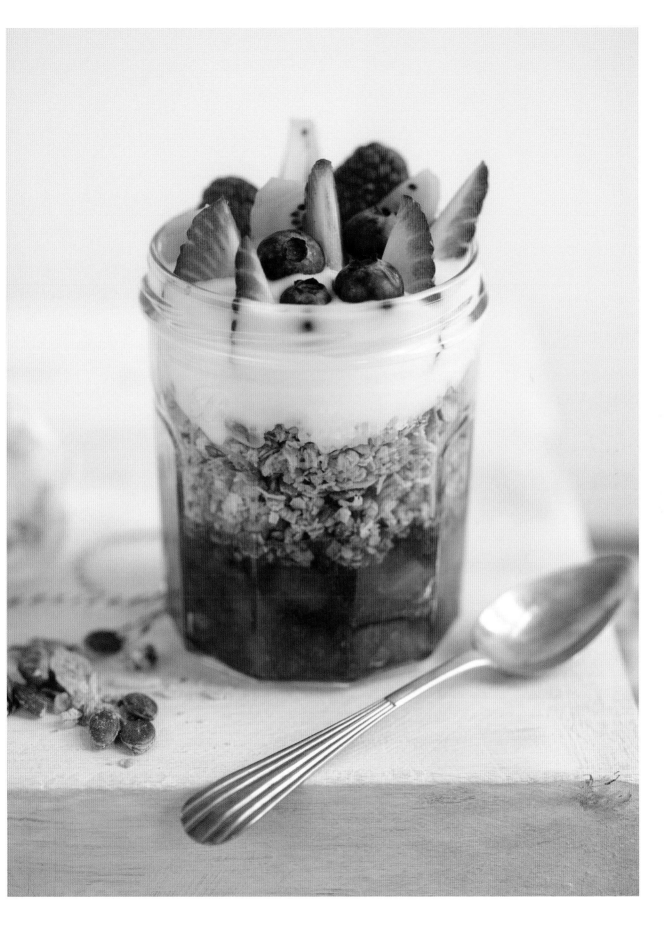

Bircher muesli

The word 'muesli' is derived from the Swiss/German word 'mues' which means to purée or mash up. Bircher Muesli was developed by a Swiss physician, Maximilian Bircher–Benner, in around 1900 as a staple food for the patients in his hospital.

It is made from whole grains, fruit, nuts and seeds mixed together, soaked overnight in water or milk, and served with yogurt.

There are some good reasons for serving a dish such as muesli for breakfast. It is low in fat, nutritionally balanced and a good source of soluble fibre that gently stimulates the bowel.

A little snack box full of Bircher muesli is easily transported and one of the best meals on-the-go you can have.

MAKES 8 SERVINGS
Hands-on time 10 minutes,
    plus 1 hour soaking

200 g/7 oz/2 cups rolled oats
60 g/2 oz/½ cup ground
    hazelnuts
4 tbsp raisins
2 tbsp seeds, such as pumpkin
    or sunflower
300 ml/10fl oz/1¼ cups almond
    milk or lactose-free milk, plus
    more if needed
200ml/7 fl oz/¾ cup water, plus
    more if needed
finely grated zest and juice
    of ½ lemon
1 walnut-sized piece of root
    ginger, very finely chopped,
    or to taste
200 ml/7 fl oz/¾ cup yogurt
200 g/7 oz/1–1½ cups fruit such
    as strawberries, raspberries
    and blueberries

Combine all the ingredients except the yogurt and fresh fruit thoroughly in a large bowl, cover and put in the fridge for 1–2 hours. Add more milk or water if you need to loosen the muesli a little.

Serve with yogurt and chopped fruit.

This will keep for up to 3 days in the fridge, but you will need to add more liquid just before serving to keep it moist.

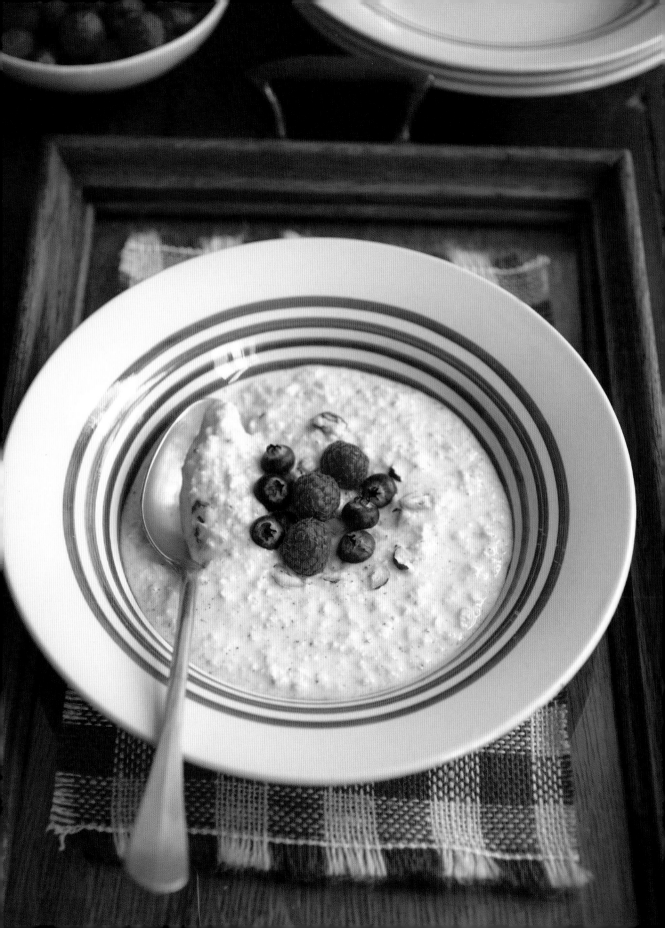

Blueberry, banana and vanilla pancakes

You would never guess these lacy, delicate pancakes contain no grains nor any type of flour. They are gluten-free and high in protein.

They are so easy and quick to make if you have a stick blender, or a liquidiser, and a non-stick frying pan. The weight and size of bananas vary considerably and it is worth weighing them before you start. A medium-sized ripe banana with its skin on weighs about 150 g/5 oz, and this is the size we have based this recipe on.

Use bananas that are ripe, but not over-ripe with black patches.

MAKES 8
Hands-on time 10 minutes
Cooking time 15 minutes

2 medium-sized ripe bananas
3 eggs
1 tsp vanilla extract
½ tsp ground cardamom seeds
  (optional)
150 g/5 oz/¾ cup blueberries
1 tbsp vegetable oil
2 tbsp maple or golden syrup
1 tsp vanilla sugar or icing
  (confectioner's) sugar

Peel the bananas and place them in a tall jug or liquidiser. Add the eggs, vanilla and ground cardamom, if using. Liquidise these ingredients and leave the batter to settle for 5 minutes. The mixture can be quite frothy at this stage and the bubbles need to disperse a little before cooking. Just before you are about to cook the pancakes, stir in 100 g/3 oz/½ cup of the blueberries.

Heat a large non-stick frying pan and, with a piece of kitchen paper, wipe oil around the pan. Pour 2 tbsp of batter into the pan for each pancake. You should be able to fit 4 small pancakes in a pan and each pancake should measure about 10 cm/4 in across.

Cook the pancakes for 2 minutes or until just set. Flip the pancakes over and cook for a further 2 minutes.

Serve the pancakes with extra blueberries, a drizzle of syrup and a dusting of vanilla sugar.

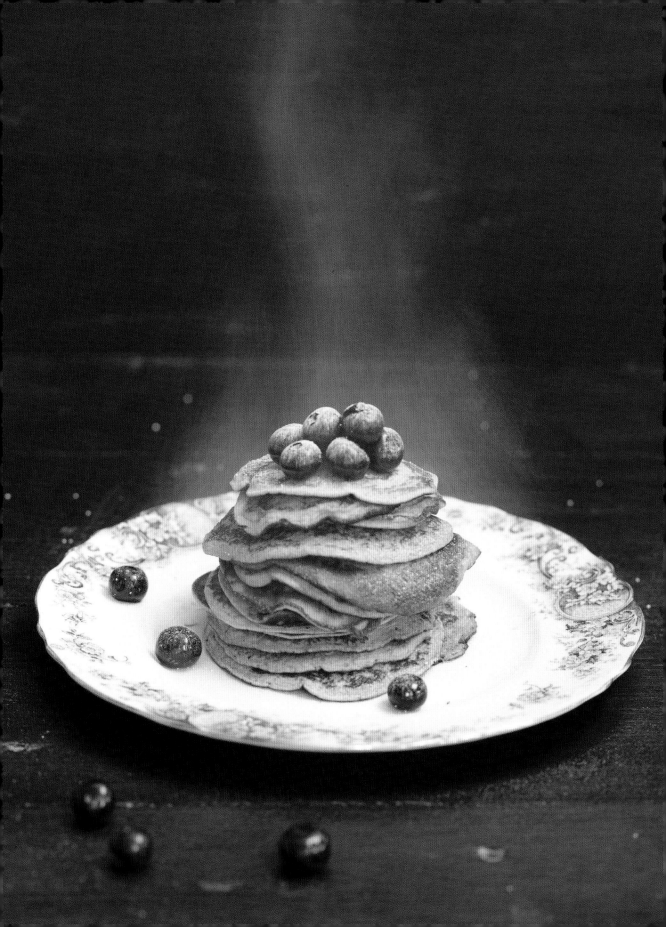

Chia seeds with raspberry sauce and cocoa nibs

Chia seed is a traditional food eaten in Central and South America. The plant bears very small white and dark brown seeds, full of short-chain omega-3 fatty acids which are converted slowly in the body into the more biologically useful long-chain omega-3 fatty acids. These are particularly important in the structure and function of nervous tissue, including the retina of the eye. A 2 tbsp serving of chia seeds should be tolerated by most people with IBS.

Both black and white chia seeds are good to eat if mixed with other ingredients, but on their own don't have much taste. Their magic is revealed when they are soaked. The seeds plump up and, like linseeds, develop a slippery coating. They slide down easily and are the kindest thing for a troubled, grumbling gut.

Chia seeds do not need any added sugar if you soak them in plant milk and serve them with fruit or a fresh fruit sauce.

SERVES 4
Hands-on time 10 minutes
Cooking time 5 minutes, plus at
   least 2 hours soaking

FOR THE CHIA SEEDS
100 g/3½ oz/⅔ cup chia seeds,
   dark or light
400 ml/¾ pint/1⅔ cups
   unsweetened lactose-free milk,
   such as soya, rice or almond
2 tsp cocoa nibs, to serve

FOR THE FRESH
   RASPBERRY SAUCE
200 g/7 oz/1½ cups raspberries
2 tbsp caster (superfine) sugar
1 tbsp lemon juice

Place the chia seeds in a bowl and add the milk. Whisk the seeds and milk together and leave to soak for 30 minutes.

To make the raspberry sauce, place the raspberries, sugar and lemon juice in a small saucepan and heat gently for about 5 minutes or until the raspberries are soft. Remove the saucepan from the heat and allow to cool a little before liquidising. Pass the sauce through a sieve if the raspberry seeds bother you. Serve with the soaked chia seeds and scatter with cocoa nibs (they have a lovely crunch and a delicious chocolate aftertaste).

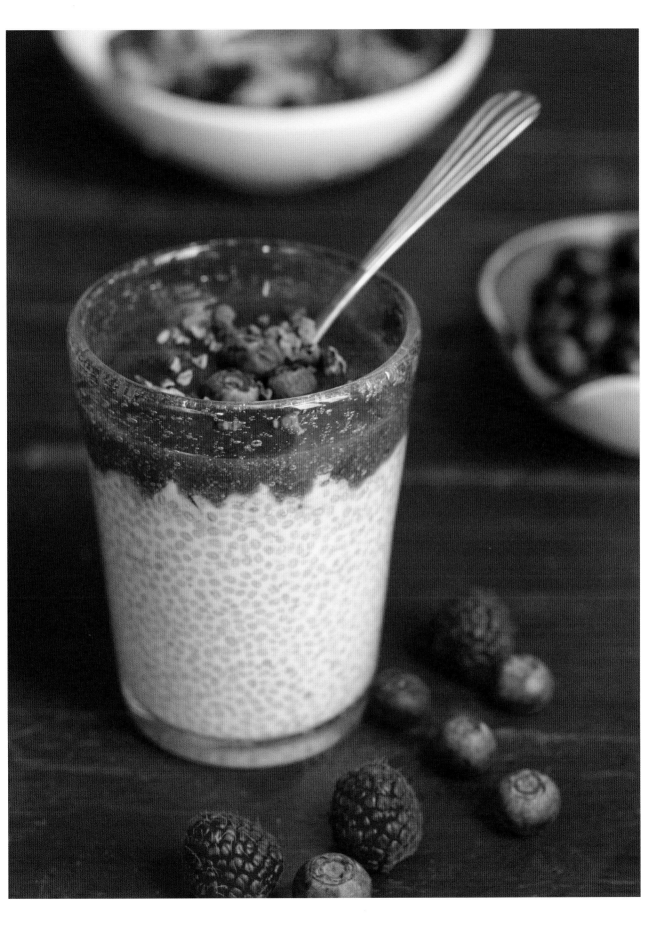

Rösti with bacon and egg

Sometimes, a cooked breakfast or brunch is just the thing to set you up for the day. It can be a colourful, sustaining, nutritionally balanced meal full of savoury flavours and an interesting array of textures. Potatoes are a good source of carbohydrate if you have problems eating bread made from wheat. Grated and made into an Alpine-style rösti, they make a good platform for bacon and eggs. This version has much less fat than most recipes for rösti and works brilliantly if you use a non-stick pan.

SERVES 4
Hands-on time 10 minutes
Cooking time 10 minutes

4 small potatoes, peeled
4 tbsp olive oil
8 rashers of lean bacon
4 eggs
a little sea salt
1 tsp vinegar

This rösti will need to be cooked in batches. Coarsely grate the potatoes into a bowl. Take handfuls of the grated potato and gently squeeze some of the moisture from them over the sink.

Heat 1 tbsp oil in a medium-sized non-stick frying pan and add about one-quarter of the grated potato. If you have a good-quality non-stick pan, you can reduce the amount of oil used to a smear. Allow the rösti to cook for a couple of minutes, then shape it into a flat cake 20 cm/8 in across, pressing down lightly with a spatula. Cook for 3–4 minutes, then gently shake the pan to loosen the rösti from the base and continue to cook until the underside is golden and crisp.

Place a plate on top of the pan and invert the pan so the rösti sits on the plate cooked-side up. Add another smear of oil to the pan and slide the potato cake back, the other way up. Cook steadily for another 5 minutes or until the underside of the rösti is crisp. Keep warm in a low oven while you cook the remaining rösti.

Meanwhile, grill the bacon for 5 minutes until crisp. Lay on kitchen paper to absorb excess fat and keep warm.

Poach the eggs: the key to a great poached egg is freshness. Fill a saucepan one-third full with cold water and bring it to the boil. Add a pinch of salt and a dash of vinegar to the water and reduce to a simmer. With a whisk, create a gentle whirlpool in the water. Crack 1 egg into a cup and gently tip into the simmering water, straight into the whirlpool. Set a timer and poach the eggs for 2 minutes for soft and 4 minutes for hard. Remove the eggs with a slotted spoon and drain on kitchen paper. (Alternatively, use an egg poacher.)

Serve the rösti with bacon and a poached egg.

Spinach and feta omelette rolls with toasted caraway seeds

Eaten plain or with a filling, omelettes are a nutritious, sustaining breakfast dish. The flavour of toasted caraway is lovely with feta, which in turn tastes really good with spinach.

Eggs are high in protein and contain a useful source of key minerals such as iodine, iron and selenium as well as all the main vitamins apart from vitamin C. Free-range organic eggs also contain the biologically useful long-chain omega-3 fatty acids, and these are the type of eggs we use.

Eggs are not associated with triggering symptoms in a sensitive gut.

SERVES 4
Hands-on time 10 minutes
Cooking time 15 minutes

FOR THE FILLING
250 g/9 oz/1 generous cup baby
    spinach leaves
120 g/4 oz/1 cup feta cheese,
    crumbled
sea salt and freshly ground
    black pepper
2 tsp caraway seeds
12 cherry tomatoes, halved

FOR THE OMELETTE
8 eggs
2 tbsp lactose-free milk
pinch of sea salt
60 g/2 oz/½ stick unsalted butter

Start with the filling. Steam the spinach for 5 minutes or until wilted. Drain carefully, taking care to remove as much moisture as you can, then chop roughly. Add the feta and a little seasoning.

Toast the caraway seeds in a hot frying pan until they begin to brown. Remove from the heat and stir the caraway seeds into the spinach mixture.

Now for the omelette. Break the eggs into a bowl, add the milk and salt and whisk thoroughly.

For each omelette, heat a little butter in a small non-stick frying pan measuring 20 cm/8 in across. When the butter has melted and begins to bubble, add one-quarter of the egg mixture and swirl it around the pan to form a circle. Cook over a low heat for 2–3 minutes until firm and golden brown underneath but with a little raw egg remaining on the top.

Spread one-quarter of the spinach filling over the middle of each omelette and scatter one-quarter of the tomato halves over that. Roll the omelette up and cut in half before serving. Repeat to cook all the omelettes.

TRY THIS:
You can add 1 tbsp of cooked quinoa to each omelette before rolling it up. This makes a more filling dish.

MAINS

It's so good to sit down to a tasty meal at the end of a day's work. So don't let your sensitive gut spoil it for you. Relax, knowing which foods you can prepare and eat with confidence.

Your main meal of the day needs to supply a balanced range of nutrients, so be sure to include a portion of cereal or other starchy food; a portion of protein from lean meat, fish, dairy or soya; some vegetables; and a portion of fruit as a dessert (see p.33). As ever, a variety of fresh ingredients not only tastes good but is more healthy.

You can personalise the recipes in this section by substituting any ingredients with reference to our guide in Gut-friendly Foods (see p.00) and your own experience. If you get in the habit of doing this, you will become a better cook and really skilled at adapting recipes to suit the sensitivities of your gut.

FISH

Fish contains important amounts of protein, essential fats, vitamins and minerals. We have used a range of readily available fish in our recipes, including smoked, canned, fresh fish and shellfish. They are all gut-friendly and provide a useful starting point for a meal cooked with potatoes, rice, quinoa, vegetables and herbs. The recipes in this section can be mixed and matched with those in the vegetarian and side dishes sections (see p.114–141).

Hot-smoked salmon with spinach and lemon

Spinach, with its dark-green, beautiful leaves, is very useful for adding to salads, wilting with fish, serving with eggs or mixing with feta cheese. It also works really well with any kind of salmon; fresh, hot-smoked or just plain smoked.

This recipe is a combination of three simple, complementary flavours. The sweetened lemon cuts through the rich salmon and the earthy spinach complements both. The hot-smoked salmon is served cold in this recipe but, if you prefer, it can be warmed.

SERVES 4
Hands-on time 10 minutes
Cooking time 3 minutes

1 lemon
2 tsp caster (superfine) sugar
2 tsp capers, drained and rinsed
2 tbsp good-quality olive oil
400 g/14 oz spinach, rinsed well
4 x 150 g/5 oz portions of
   hot-smoked salmon
sea salt and freshly ground
   black pepper

Peel the skin and pith from the lemon. Slice the flesh thinly and remove any pips. Place the lemon, any excess juice, caster sugar, capers and olive oil in a bowl and mix well. Set aside.

Cook the spinach in a saucepan for a couple of minutes with 2 tbsp of water, or steam it over boiling water. Turn the spinach leaves with tongs halfway through cooking and cook until the leaves are wilted. Drain in a colander and squeeze excess moisture from the leaves.

Divide the spinach between 4 plates and place a portion of salmon on top of each. Place a little sliced lemon to one side and dress the salmon and spinach with the remaining lemon juice, capers and olive oil, seasoning well. This dish works well served with Lemon rice with coriander and mustard seeds (see p.136) or plain basmati.

Baked white fish with crunchy pine nut, Parmesan and basil crust

A flavoured breadcrumb crust can transform a humble piece of fish into a first-class tasty dish. Always use really fresh fish if you can get it. As for breadcrumbs, you can use gluten-free or sourdough if you prefer, but you should be comfortable with small quantities of one-day-old white bread (one slice per person).

This would be delicious with Fennel and potato gratin (see p.138).

SERVES 4
Hands-on time 10 minutes
Cooking time 10 minutes

40 g/1½ oz/⅓cup pine nuts,
    slightly crushed
100 g/4 oz/1 cup fresh white
    breadcrumbs
4 tbsp Parmesan cheese,
    finely grated
4 tbsp chopped basil leaves
sea salt and freshly ground
    black pepper
3 tbsp olive oil
4 x 120 g/4 oz white fish fillets,
    such as cod, haddock or hake
2 tbsp white wine

Preheat the oven to 200°C/400°F/gas 6.

Mix together the pine nuts, breadcrumbs, Parmesan, basil, seasoning and 2 tbsp of the olive oil in a small bowl.

Remove any pin bones from the fish and rinse under cold water. Pat the fillets dry with kitchen paper.

Brush an ovenproof dish with the remaining olive oil. Lay the fish fillets in the dish and sprinkle with the wine. Cover with the breadcrumbs and cook for about 10 minutes, or until the topping is golden brown and crunchy.

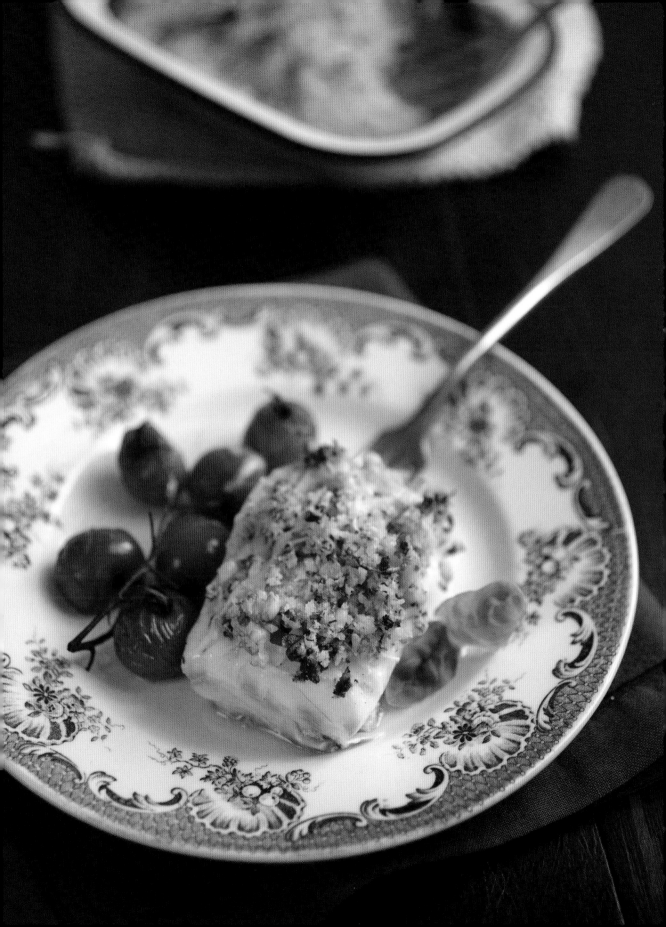

Salmon, quinoa and crispy potato salad with a blueberry and maple syrup dressing

We really encourage you to give this a try. You do not have to use all the ingredients listed for it to taste fabulous. You can adapt it according to taste and with reference to the list of gut-friendly ingredients (see p.30). We love to forage for wild foods in hedgerows and we included some hazelnuts we found in this recipe. Hazelnuts add essential fatty acids, proteins and energy, and can be eaten in moderation by people with a sensitive gut.

SERVES 4

Hands-on time 15 minutes

Cooking time 45 minutes

FOR THE SALAD

200 g/7 oz new potatoes, rinsed

1–2 tbsp olive oil

sea salt and ground black pepper

60 g/2 oz/⅓ cup quinoa

300 g/10 oz salmon

4 handfuls of watercress and
    rocket (arugula) leaves

leaves of 1 head of red chicory

¼ cucumber, halved and sliced

4 spring onions (scallions), green
    leaves only

2 tbsp canned lentils, drained
    and rinsed well

micro salad leaves, such as purple
    radish or cress (optional)

1 tbsp shelled hazelnuts
    (optional)

FOR THE DRESSING

100 g/3½ oz/½ cup blueberries

3 tbsp olive oil

1 tbsp lemon juice

1 tbsp maple syrup

Preheat the oven to 200°C/400°F/gas 6.

Steam the potatoes until tender, then cool and cut in half. Using a potato masher, crush the potatoes slightly and place in a roasting tin with the olive oil, mixing well. Sprinkle with a little salt and cook for about 30 minutes until crisp and golden brown.

Meanwhile, cook the quinoa in boiling water for 10 minutes, or according to the packet instructions, then drain.

Place the salmon on a sheet of foil, season well and fold the foil into an envelope. Place the salmon in a roasting tin and cook for 10 minutes. Remove from the oven and leave to cool, then flake the fish.

To make the dressing, crush half the blueberries in a mortar and pestle and add the olive oil, lemon juice and maple syrup. Season with a little salt and pepper and mix well.

Place the leaves, cucumber and spring onions on a serving dish. Arrange the potatoes on the salad, with the salmon. Sprinkle with the quinoa and lentils and dress with the dressing. Scatter the remaining blueberries over the salad together with any micro herbs or nuts.

TRY THIS:
Use smoked trout instead of salmon.

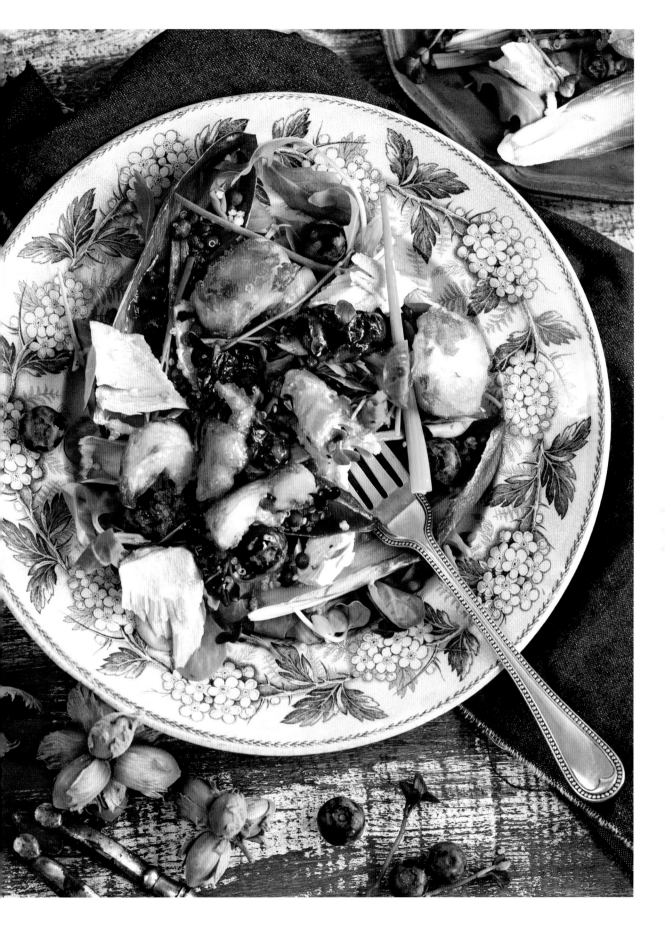

Fish pie with two-potato mash

Getting home hungry and putting delicious food on the table can be a challenge and it's often tempting to try ready-made frozen dishes, but they are not always convenient or tasty. The cooking times from frozen can be more than it would take you to prepare the dish from scratch. This is a beautiful classic fish pie. It is easy to make and looks and tastes great. That said, it makes sense to cook one of these pies for supper and freeze a spare if you can; it will keep for up to three months. (Open-freeze the fish pie before cooking, then wrap in foil or cling film/plastic wrap. Defrost in the fridge the night before it is needed and cook as in the recipe.)

SERVES 6
Hands-on time 20 minutes
Cooking time 40 minutes

FOR THE FILLING
400 ml/14 fl oz/1⅓ cups lactose-
    free milk
green leaves of 2 young leeks
1 bay leaf
1 tsp black peppercorns
25 g/1 oz/2 tbsp unsalted butter
2 tbsp plain flour or cornflour
    (cornstarch)
4 tbsp dry white wine
1 tbsp crème fraîche (optional)
1 tbsp chopped parsley leaves
sea salt and ground black pepper
500 g/18 oz mixed fish in large
    chunks, such as cod, smoked
    haddock or salmon

FOR THE TOPPING
1 small sweet potato, peeled and
    cut into large chunks
2 large white potatoes, peeled
    and cut into large chunks
2–3 tbsp lactose-free milk
25 g/1 oz/2 tbsp unsalted butter
25 g/1 oz/¼ cup Gruyère, grated

To make the filling, pour the milk into a large saucepan. Add the leek leaves, bay leaf and peppercorns and bring to a gentle simmer over a low heat. Remove from the heat and leave to stand for 20 minutes to infuse. Strain through a colander into a jug.

Melt the butter in a medium-sized saucepan and stir in the flour or cornflour. Cook for a few seconds, adding first the wine, then, gradually, the flavoured milk, stirring constantly. Simmer for 3–4 minutes until it becomes smooth and glossy. Add the crème fraîche (if using) and parsley, taste and season carefully.

Spoon half the sauce into an ovenproof dish. Scatter the fish over, then pour the remaining sauce over the fish.

To make the topping, cover the potatoes with water and bring to the boil, then reduce the heat and simmer for 15 minutes or until really soft. Preheat the oven to 200°C/400°F/gas 6.

Drain the potatoes and return to the pan. Use a potato ricer or potato masher to mash the potatoes. Add enough milk to loosen them so you can spread them over the fish. Mix in the butter and season to taste. Spread the mash over the filling and sprinkle the cheese over the top.

Bake in the oven for 40 minutes until golden brown and the sauce is bubbling through the topping.

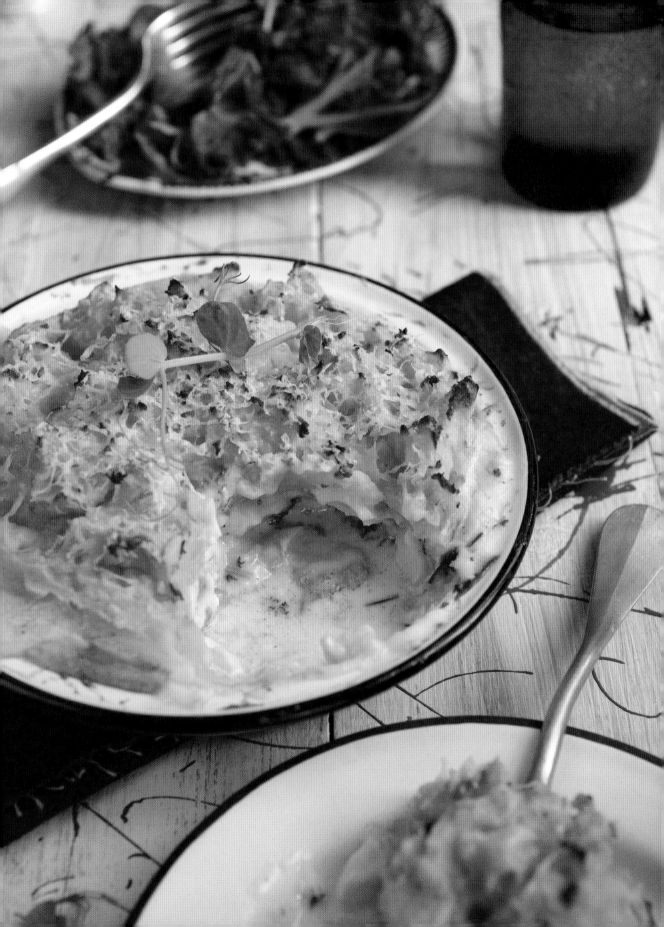

Brill with green bean and watercress salad

Green beans and white fish go together really well. Most people like green beans and they are usually available year round. They are a great vegetable if you have a sensitive gut, because they are low in fermentable carbohydrates and contain a useful amount of fibre. This is a lovely, nutritionally balanced meal, which is also low in fat. You can also substitute the brill for cod or any other white fish.

SERVES 4
Hands-on time 10 minutes
Cooking time 15 minutes

2 large potatoes, peeled and
   thinly sliced
sea salt and freshly ground
   black pepper
150 g/5 oz/1 cup green beans,
   topped and tailed
handful of watercress, coarse
   stalks removed
8 radishes, quartered
5 x 150 g/5 oz brill fillets, skin on,
   pin bones removed
1 tbsp olive oil,
   plus more for the potatoes

FOR THE DRESSING
3 tbsp olive oil
1 tbsp lemon juice

Cook the potatoes in a pan of salted boiling water for 5 minutes, then drain and set aside.

Blanch the green beans in a small saucepan of boiling water for 5 minutes until tender. Drain and plunge into a bowl of cold water to keep them crisp and retain their colour.

To make the dressing, whisk together the olive oil with the lemon juice and a little salt and pepper.

Combine the green beans, watercress and radishes, and add the dressing. Toss the salad so it is well coated with the dressing.

Heat a non-stick frying pan over a high heat and rub both sides of the fish with olive oil. Place in the pan skin-side down and cook for about 5 minutes until crisp. Turn the fillets over and cook for a further 2 minutes or until the centre of the fillets is just opaque. Keep the fish warm for a couple of minutes.

Drizzle a little olive oil in a separate frying pan over a medium heat and sauté the potato slices, taking care not to break them up. Divide the potatoes and salad between 4 plates and top with the fish.

TRY THIS:
• Substitute any white fish, such as hake, halibut or cod.
• Use sliced new potatoes rather than floury potatoes.

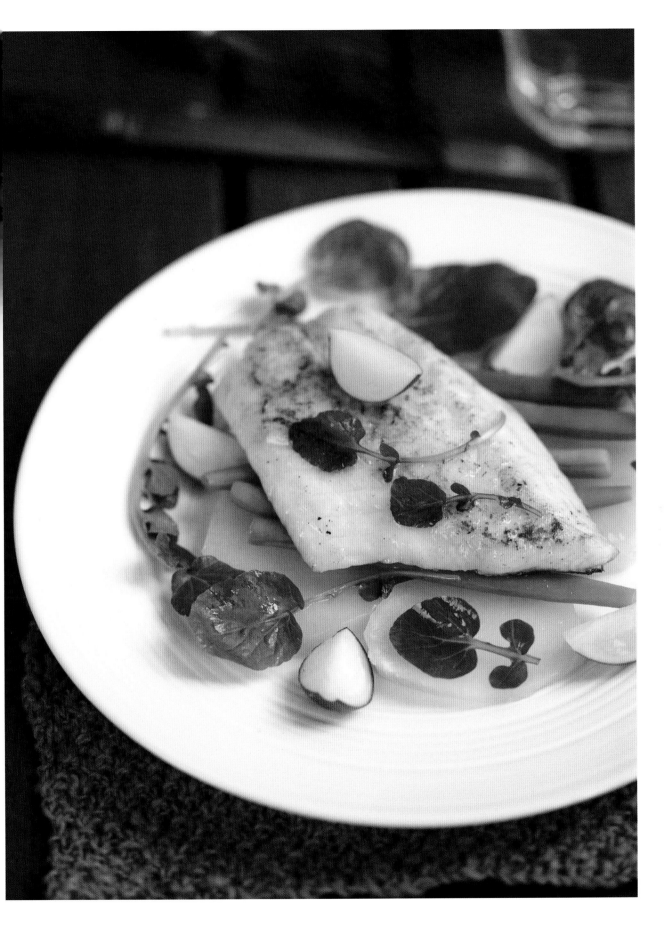

Courgetti with puttanesca sauce

This dish is so quick to prepare and has such piquant, salty, gutsy flavours. The puttanesca sauce is mixed with courgetti, made by spiralizing courgette to make long strips that look like spaghetti. (If you don't have a spiralizer, you can create a similar effect with a julienne peeler or a regular potato peeler.)

Most people can tolerate 75 g/3 oz/1½ cups of cooked spaghetti in a sitting. If this is not enough to satisfy hunger, it can be mixed with a portion of buckwheat or rice noodles. They both taste good with Italian flavours, even though they aren't usually associated with them.

SERVES 4
Hands-on time 10 minutes
Cooking time 10 minutes

2 courgettes (zucchini), ends cut
    off, halved
2 tbsp olive oil
1 garlic clove, sliced
150 g/5 oz/1 cup spaghetti,
    buckwheat or rice noodles
8 anchovy fillets, roughly
    chopped
150 g/5 oz/scant 1 cup pitted
    black olives, roughly chopped
1 tbsp capers, rinsed and
    roughly chopped
1 large beef tomato (beefsteak
    tomato), chopped
freshly ground black pepper
60 g/2 oz/⅔ cup Parmesan
    cheese, finely grated
a few basil leaves, to serve

Using a spiralizer or julienne cutter, make long strips from the courgette. This is the courgetti.

Drizzle the base of a large non-stick saucepan with olive oil and gently fry the garlic until it begins to brown. Remove the garlic from the oil and discard.

Add the courgetti to the saucepan and cook gently in the garlic-infused oil for 5 minutes.

At this point, cook the spaghetti or noodles according to the packet instructions.

Add the anchovies, olives, capers and tomato to the courgetti, increase the heat a little and cook for a further 5 minutes.

Drain the pasta, reserving a little of the cooking water, and mix with the courgetti and sauce. Add a little of the cooking water to loosen the sauce a little if you need to. Taste the sauce, adjust the seasoning with pepper if required, and scatter with the Parmesan and torn basil leaves.

TRY THIS:
You can vary this recipe by substituting Pesto (see p.48) for the puttanesca sauce.

Herby fish cakes in tomato sauce

This is a delicious recipe and, if you want to make it ahead, you can freeze the uncooked fish cakes. Paprika is not usually hot, but smoked paprika can be, so make sure it is not labelled as 'hot' or 'piccante' on the label. If it is, substitute it with unsmoked paprika. The paprika adds a beautiful brick-red tone to this dish and a smoky flavour. These fish cakes go really well with Lemon rice with coriander and mustard seeds (see p.136).

SERVES 4–6

Hands-on time 20 minutes

Cooking time 35 minutes,
    plus 30 minutes chilling

FOR THE FISH CAKES

400 g/14 oz white fish

sea salt and ground black pepper

1 tbsp chopped parsley leaves

1 tbsp chopped coriander (cilantro)

1 tbsp chopped chives

2 tsp ground cumin

1 slice of white bread, made into
    breadcrumbs

1 egg, lightly beaten

zest and juice of 1 lemon

olive oil

FOR THE TOMATO SAUCE

1 tbsp olive oil

1 garlic clove, sliced

1 celery stalk, finely chopped

1 tbsp chopped chives

1 tbsp ground cumin

150 ml/5 fl oz/⅔ cup white wine

400 g/14 oz can plum tomatoes

½ tsp smoked paprika

½ tsp sugar

2 bay leaves

sea salt and ground black pepper

1 tbsp chopped parsley or
    coriander (cilantro) leaves

For the fish cakes, chop the fish finely and place in a bowl with all the other ingredients apart from the lemon juice and olive oil. Mix well. Use your hands shape the mixture into compact fish cakes 3 cm/1½ in thick and 8 cm/3 in wide. This amount of mixture should make 8 fish cakes. Place them on a plate, cover with cling film (plastic wrap) and refrigerate for 30 minutes to firm up. (They can be frozen at this stage for use later.)

To make the sauce, pour the oil into a large non-stick saucepan and warm gently. Add the garlic to the oil and cook until just turning brown. Discard the garlic.

Add the celery, chives and cumin to the garlic-flavoured oil and sweat for 3 minutes or until the celery is soft. Add the wine and increase the heat to allow it to evaporate. Add the canned tomatoes, smoked paprika, sugar and bay leaves. Simmer for 15 minutes until it is quite thick and the tomatoes have broken down to a pulp. Taste and season the sauce with salt and pepper. Stir in a little water if it looks too thick.

Heat a drizzle of olive oil in a non-stick pan and sear the fish cakes on each side for about 3 minutes until they just begin to colour. Place the seared fish cakes in the tomato sauce; they need to be half submerged. Place a lid on the saucepan and simmer the fish cakes for 15 minutes. Serve sprinkled with a little chopped coriander or parsley and a squeeze of lemon juice.

Prawn laksa

Laksa is a Malaysian noodle soup with a fragrant coconut broth flavoured with fish sauce, ginger and lime. This dish will warm you through to your soul and is gentle on the gut. Kaffir lime leaves add zest to this dish; they can be found in some supermarkets, Thai and Asian food shops, but if you can't find them, don't worry, the laksa will still taste good.

SERVES 4

Hands-on time 20 minutes

Cooking time 15 minutes

1 tbsp rapeseed or other
  flavourless oil
280 g/10 oz/2 cups sweet potato,
  peeled and cut into
  2 cm (1 in) cubes
3 spring onions (scallions), green
  leaves only, sliced
1 tbsp grated root ginger
200 ml/7 fl oz/1 cup coconut milk
1 tbsp fish sauce
2 kaffir lime leaves
pinch of vegetable stock powder
  (optional)
6 water chestnuts, sliced
juice and finely grated zest
  of ½ lime
150 g/5 oz/1 cup raw tiger
  prawns (jumbo shrimp)
1 head of pak choi, sliced
1 tbsp chopped coriander
  (cilantro) leaves, plus
  more to serve
sea salt and freshly ground
  black pepper
soy sauce, to taste
150 g/5 oz/1 cup rice noodles,
  cooked according to the
  packet instructions

Warm a little oil in a large wok, add the sweet potato and cook until soft and beginning to brown. Throw in the spring onion tops and ginger, and cook for about 1 minute.

Pour the coconut milk and the same amount of water into the wok, then add the fish sauce and lime leaves. Bring the liquid to a gentle boil. Add the stock powder, if using, and stir well before adding the water chestnuts, lime zest, prawns and pak choi. Cook the laksa for 5 minutes.

Finish the laksa by adding the coriander and lime juice, tasting as you go. Adjust the seasoning and add a little soy sauce if you need extra flavour.

Place a swirl of noodles in each of 4 bowls, pour over the laksa, and finish with a few chopped coriander leaves.

TRY THIS:

• *Substitute the prawns with shreds of raw chicken, white fish or salmon.*
• *Add more vegetables, or tofu, for a vegetarian version.*

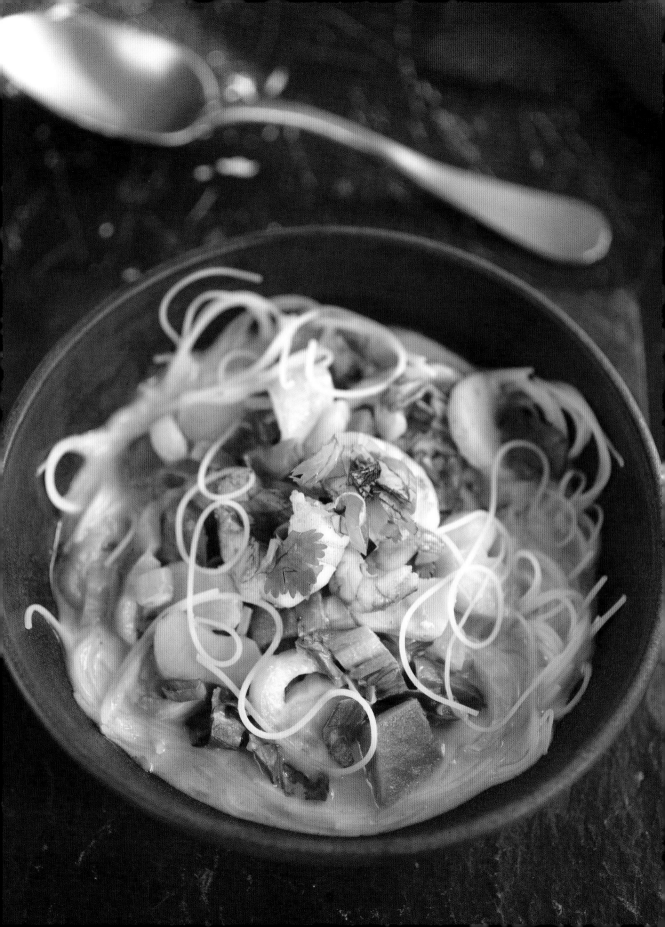

Red peppers with anchovies and tomatoes

These slow-cooked peppers are great as a small, tasty meal or snack and can be cooked very quickly in a cast-iron pan (or a small roasting tin) placed in a hot oven.

As the peppers cook, their flavours mingle with those of anchovies, garlic oil and tomatoes to form a piquant syrup that can be mopped up with pieces of Spelt sourdough bread (see p.54) or a portion of wet polenta.

SERVES 4
Hands-on time 5 minutes
Cooking time 40 minutes

4 red (bell) peppers
2 tbsp Garlic-infused oil (see p.36), or olive oil
50 g/2 oz can anchovy fillets, chopped
6 tomatoes, chopped
freshly ground black pepper
basil leaves, to serve
30 g/1 oz/⅓ cup Parmesan cheese, grated
freshly ground black pepper
150 g/5 oz/1 cup rice noodles, cooked according to the packet instructions

Preheat the oven to 200°C/400°F/gas 6.

Cut the peppers in half lengthways and remove the seeds. Leave the stalks on as they look good and help to keep their structure.

Lay the pepper halves in a lightly oiled roasting tin or cast-iron pan. Place one-eighth of the chopped anchovies and tomatoes in each. Drizzle with the remaining oil and season with pepper.

Cook for 45 minutes, or until the peppers are tender and running with tomato- and anchovy-flavoured juices. Serve with torn basil leaves and a sprinkling of grated Parmesan cheese. This would be lovely with buckwheat noodles or plain risotto.

TRY THIS:
Add black or green olives to the peppers as they cook.

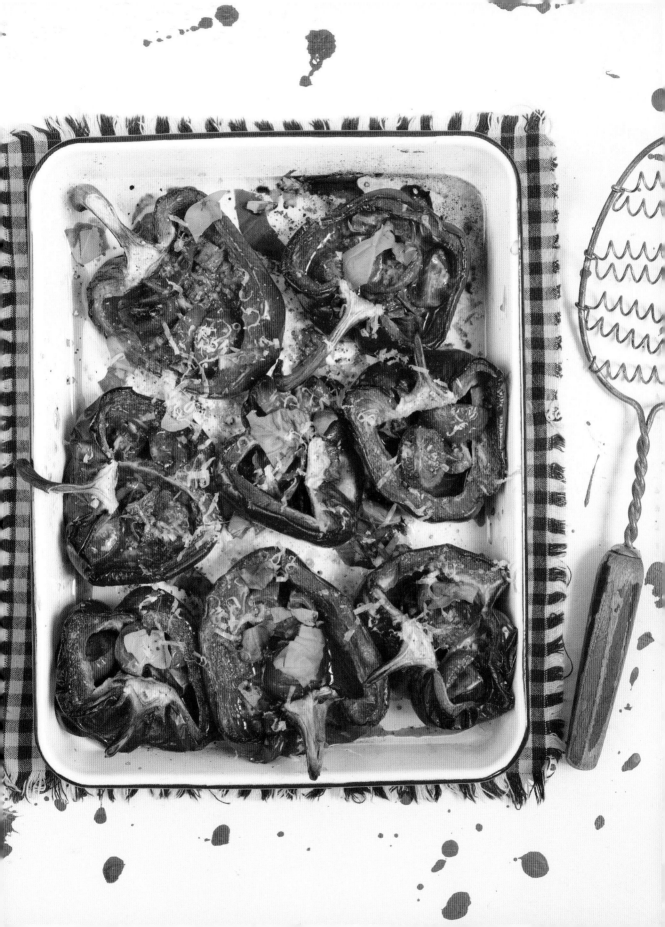

Cod parcels with sauce vierge

This can be made with any thick steak of fish such as cod, tuna, shark or swordfish.

Sauce vierge is tangy, colourful and full of flavour. It is perfect with white fish and normally contains a few mild-flavoured, finely chopped shallots. In this recipe, we have substituted a few chives to make it more soothing to eat.

This would be delicious with Oven-baked potatoes with rosemary and garlic oil (see p.141) and a bowl of steamed vegetables.

SERVES 4
Hands-on time 10 minutes
Cooking time 10 minutes

FOR THE FISH
4 x 150 g/5 oz fillets of cod,
   checked for pin bones
4 tbsp dry white wine
sea salt and freshly ground
   black pepper
4 sprigs of parsley or dill

FOR THE SAUCE VIERGE
100 ml/3½ fl oz/½ cup extra-
   virgin olive oil
juice of ½ lemon
1 large tomato, skinned
   and chopped
2 tbsp capers, drained and
   rinsed, chopped if large
1 tbsp finely chopped basil leaves
1 tbsp finely chopped
   parsley leaves
½ tbsp finely chopped chives
sea salt and freshly ground
   black pepper

Preheat the oven to 200°C/400°F/gas 6.

Place 4 squares of foil, each measuring 25 cm/10 in, on 2 baking trays. Place each piece of fish in the centre of a piece of foil.

Sprinkle the fish with the wine and season with salt and pepper. Place a sprig of parsley or dill on each piece of fish and seal the parcel by folding around the edges of the foil.

Cook for 10 minutes. Unwrap one of the parcels and check the fish is cooked. It should look firm and the flesh should be white.

To prepare the sauce vierge, whisk the olive oil and lemon juice in a small bowl. Add the tomato and the remaining ingredients and mix well. Season with salt and pepper, and taste the sauce to check the balance of flavours is to your liking.

Serve each fish parcel on a plate with a bowl of sauce vierge for everyone to share.

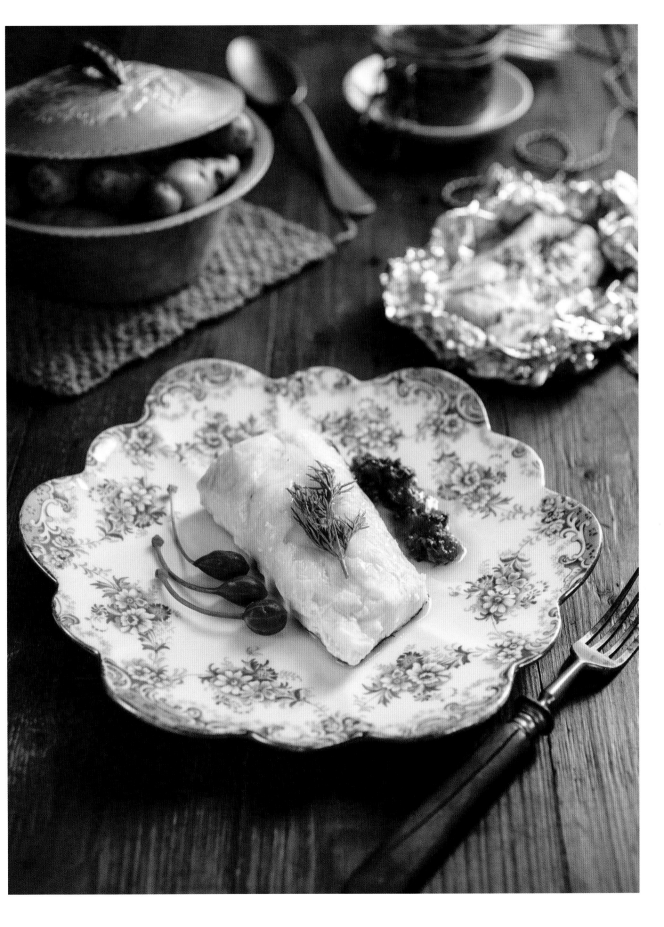

Spiced haddock chowder

Chowder is a classic New England fish stew cooked with milk and thickened with potatoes. It is a quick, flavoursome dish made from humble ingredients that feel comforting and are nutritious. The key to making this dish taste fantastic is to cook each stage carefully.

SERVES 4
Hands-on time 10 minutes
Cooking time 50 minutes

4 x 150 g/5 oz portions undyed
   smoked haddock, skinned
   and boned
500 ml/18 fl oz/2 cups lactose-
   free milk
1 bay leaf
1 tsp black peppercorns
20 g/¾ oz/1½ tbsp unsalted
   butter
½ tsp turmeric
200 g/7 oz /²⁄₃ cup swede
   (Swedish/yellow turnip),
   finely chopped
1 carrot, finely chopped
1 large potato, finely chopped
green leaves of 4 young leeks,
   finely sliced
sea salt and freshly ground
   black pepper
1 tbsp chopped parsley leaves

Place the haddock fillet in a large saucepan with the milk, bay leaf and peppercorns. Bring to a simmer and turn off the heat. Place a lid on the saucepan and leave to infuse for up to 30 minutes.

Melt the butter in a large, lidded non-stick saucepan or frying pan and add the turmeric, swede, carrot, potato and leeks. Shake the pan around a little to ensure the vegetables are well coated in butter and place a lid on. Sweat the vegetables for about 5 minutes or until soft.

Strain the haddock and reserve the milk, taking care to remove the peppercorns and bay leaf.

Add the infused milk to the vegetables and continue to cook gently over a low heat for about 10 minutes. Remove a few of the potato pieces from the pan, crush them, then return them to the pan to thicken the sauce a little.

Place the haddock on top of the vegetables, return the lid to the pan and allow to cook for about 5 minutes. Season the chowder and scatter the parsley over to serve.

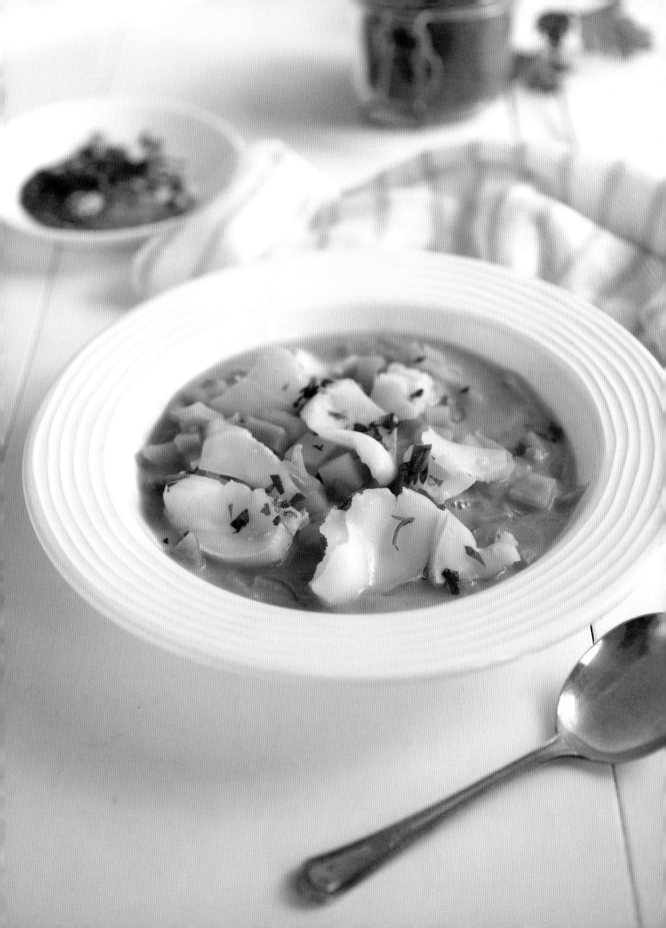

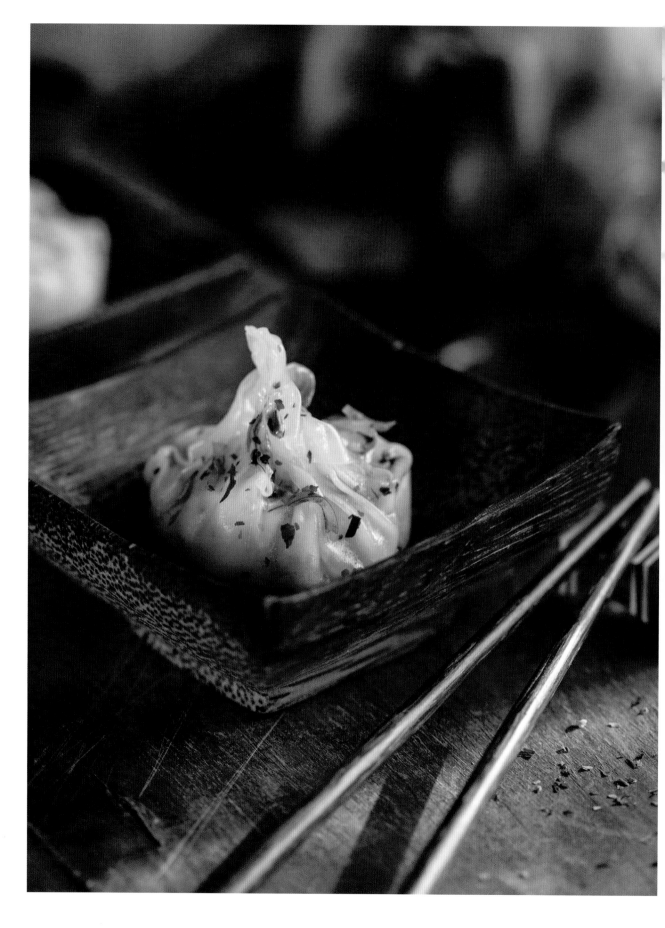

Thai-flavoured fish in rice purses

A light meal luxuriant in the gentle soothing flavours of lemongrass, ginger and coconut. The fragrant fish mixture is wrapped in rice flour pancakes pulled together at the top like a purse. The delightful little parcels are delicious dipped into the seaweed-flavoured dressing and served with steamed basmati rice and vegetables such as steamed pak choi.

This well-balanced meal should make you feel wonderful, as it is delicious but light and soothing.

SERVES 4

Hands-on time 20 minutes

Cooking time 5 minutes,
    plus 30 minutes infusing

FOR THE DRESSING

2 tbsp rice wine vinegar

5 tbsp soy sauce

2 tbsp sesame oil

green leaves of 1 spring onion
    (scallion), finely chopped

¼ mild red chilli, finely chopped
    (optional)

1 sheet nori

FOR THE FISH

400 g/14 oz fillet of white fish,
    such as cod, haddock or hake

green leaves from 4 spring onions
    (scallions), finely chopped

1 lemongrass stalk, outer leaves
    removed, finely chopped

2 tsp sesame oil

1 tbsp Garlic-infused oil (see
    p.36)

2 tsp fish sauce

2 cm/1 in root ginger, peeled and
    grated

4 tbsp coconut milk

2 tsp cornflour (cornstarch)

16 rice flour pancakes

To make the dressing, whisk the vinegar, soy sauce and sesame oil in a bowl. Add the spring onion leaves and finely chopped chilli, if using. Crumble the nori into the dressing and give a final mix. Leave the dressing to infuse for 30 minutes. Divide it into small bowls to be served at the table.

To make the fish purses, remove the skin from the fish and check for any stray bones. Chop it into 1 cm/½ in cubes and mix with all the other ingredients except the pancakes.

Take 2 clean, wet tea towels. Place the pancakes on one and cover with the other. Leave for 10 minutes, then uncover. The rice pancakes should now be soft and pliable.

Place a little of the fish mixture into the centre of each of the pancakes and then draw the edges of the pancake together to make a purse. Place in a steamer over a pan of gently boiling water and steam for 5 minutes.

Dip the fish purses into the dressing to eat.

Spelt sourdough pizza with anchovies

If you master the art of making spelt breads (see p.52) you may want other dishes to make with the dough. Spelt dough is ideal for pizza and you can customise the topping to whatever suits you.

There are a few things to know about making great pizza at home. Preheat the oven in good time. Pizza needs searing heat to cook well. Roll the dough thin so, when the pizza is cooked, the rim is crisp and the centre remains slightly soft. Use a good, thick tomato sauce on the base but, if you are short of time, use thinly sliced ripe tomatoes which have enough flavour once roasted in the oven.

Less is more with regard to toppings. Use three or four well-chosen complementary toppings rather than trying to put everything on your pizza. Choose ingredients full of umami flavours: we have included anchovies and olives, but you could also use Parma ham or chorizo. Try to keep to a theme for your pizza. Think of the pizza base as something that needs dressing up tastefully. If you load too many toppings on, the middle will remain uncooked and soggy. Soggy is bad.

SERVES 4
Hands-on time 1 hour
Cooking time 15 minutes

300 g/10 oz Spelt sourdough or
    Overnight white dough (see
    p.52 and p.54)
spelt flour, to dust
1 quantity Basic tomato sauce
    (see p.46)
sea salt and ground black pepper
1 tsp dried oregano
3 tbsp Garlic-infused oil (see
    p.36) or olive oil
2 medium courgettes (zucchini),
    sliced lengthways into 5 strips
    (add the flower if you have it)
2 handfuls of green beans
50 g/2 oz can of anchovies
100 g/3 oz/½ cup black olives
2 x 125 g/4 oz balls mozzarella,
    drained and torn into pieces
handful of rocket (arugula)

Preheat the oven to 230°C/450°F/gas 8. Divide the bread dough into 4. Place each on a piece of non-stick baking parchment dusted with spelt flour and roll into a circle 30 cm/12 in across and 0.5 cm/¼ in thick.

Top with a thin layer of tomato sauce and sprinkle with salt, pepper and oregano. Drizzle with oil and place in the oven to cook for 10 minutes. Meanwhile, daub the courgette with a little olive oil and griddle until almost cooked. Steam the green beans for 5 minutes.

When the pizzas are almost cooked, remove them from the oven and arrange the toppings over (not the rocket yet), placing pieces of mozzarella over the top.

Return the pizza to the searing-hot oven for another 5–10 minutes until the edges are crisp and well browned.

Remove from the oven, cut into pieces and serve strewn with rocket, eating with your fingers as is traditional in Italy.

TRY THIS:
Replace the anchovies with roasted red peppers or grilled aubergines (eggplants) to make it vegetarian.

Smoked salmon and lemon risotto

This is one of our favourite risottos. Limonene is the aromatic oil present in the skin of lemons and it really lifts the flavour here.

This risotto can be made without goat's cheese, but a sprinkle of grated Parmesan to finish is always lovely.

If you can, make your own stock without onions (see p.44), but otherwise use a dilute organic stock and bolster the other flavours in the dish with wine, judicious seasoning, herbs and a generous sprinkle of Parmesan.

SERVES 4
Hands-on time 5 minutes
Cooking time 20 minutes

green leaves from 4 spring onions
    (scallions) or 1 leek
1 celery stalk, finely chopped
2 tbsp olive oil
300 g/10 oz/1½ cups risotto rice
1 small glass (150 ml/5 fl oz/⅔
    cup) dry white wine or
    vermouth
1 litre/1¾ pints/1 quart warm,
    home-made Vegetable stock
    (see p.44)
80 g/3 oz/¼ cup soft goat's
    cheese
a few sprigs of lemon thyme,
    leaves picked
finely grated zest and juice
    of 1 lemon
150 g/5 oz smoked salmon, cut
    into strips
100 g/3 oz rocket (arugula)
sea salt and freshly ground
    black pepper
60 g/2 oz/⅔ cup Parmesan
    cheese, finely grated

Sweat the spring onion/leek leaves and celery in half the oil for 5 minutes, or until soft. Add the rice and continue to cook for 5 minutes until it just begins to toast.

Add the wine and allow this to evaporate before gradually adding the warm stock a ladle at a time, allowing it to evaporate before adding more. Stir the risotto continuously with a wooden spoon until the rice is soft but still has a slight bite (this should take about 20 minutes). Add the goat's cheese, lemon thyme, lemon zest and juice to taste, reserving a little lemon juice. Stir the smoked salmon through.

Dress the rocket with a sprinkle of sea salt, the reserved lemon juice and a drizzle of olive oil.

Serve the risotto with the dressed rocket and grated Parmesan cheese.

TRY THIS:
Replace the smoked salmon and goat's cheese with:
* *smoked haddock and a handful of spinach*
* *smoky bacon, ham and shaving of fennel*
* *strips of roast pepper and a handful of grated hard goat's cheese*
* *young vegetables such as carrots and courgette.*

MEAT

Meat contains important amounts of protein, essential fats, vitamins and minerals. Red meats such as beef, lamb and pork are often high in fat, so it is best to choose leaner cuts and to serve a small portion size, or use more of the less fatty meats, such as chicken.

You may like to serve interesting side dishes (see pp.136–141) with these meat recipes, or team them with our vegetarian recipes (see pp.114–135).

Smoked bacon, kale and crispy potatoes

Any kind of pork goes really well with any kind of cabbage. In this recipe, kale is wilted in a head of steam and retains the colour of its frilly, dark-green leaves. This is a simple, nutritious meal that you can put together really quickly and add other ingredients if you fancy. A poached egg on top might be nice.

SERVES 4
Hands-on time 10 minutes
Cooking time 15 minutes

250 g/9 oz/3 cups curly kale
200 g/7 oz/1 cup potato, peeled and cut into 2 cm/1 in cubes
8 rashers of smoked, dry-cured back bacon, fat trimmed, cut into 2 cm/1 in strips
½ tbsp groundnut or sunflower oil
sea salt and freshly ground black pepper

Wash the kale thoroughly and remove the thick ribs in the centre of the leaves. Place the leaves on top of each other and shred using a sharp knife.

Steam the potatoes for about 5 minutes until just soft. Remove the potatoes from the steamer and set aside.

Warm a non-stick pan on the hob and gently fry the bacon until golden brown. Remove from the pan. Add a drizzle of oil to the pan and add the cooked potatoes. Sauté until crisp and golden brown.

Steam the kale for a couple of minutes so it 'relaxes'; it should just flop in the pan. Drain the kale, place it on a serving plate and scatter with the crisp, cooked bacon and potatoes. Sprinkle with a little salt and pepper.

Chicken with green olives and smoked paprika

Joan says: 'I have been making this since I was a student. A Spanish friend made it for a crowded table and everyone loved the smell of it cooking and the exciting mix of flavours. I was always struck by how she fried the garlic in oil and then removed it from the pan, because by the time garlic browns it has lost its flavour to the oil and can taste bitter. It was a useful tip.'

The dish works well because the slow cooking yields rich-tasting gravy which is flavoured by olives and smoked paprika.

This is another great one-pot meal with both meat and vegetables included. Any left over can be eaten the following day.

SERVES 6–8
Hands-on time 20 minutes
Cooking time 1 hour

4 tbsp olive oil
2 garlic cloves, peeled and sliced
1 x 2 kg/4 lb chicken, jointed,
   or 8 chicken thighs
sea salt and freshly ground
   black pepper
2 large floury potatoes, peeled,
   cut into 5 cm/2 in chunks
4 large carrots, peeled, cut into
   thick rings
270 g/10 oz jar of queen (large
   green) olives with stones
1 bay leaf
1 tsp sweet smoked paprika
2 tsp sweet paprika
1 tbsp chopped parsley leaves
1 tbsp chopped parsley or
   coriander (cilantro) leaves,
   to serve

Warm the olive oil in a large non-stick frying pan and gently cook the garlic. When the garlic begins to brown, remove from the saucepan and discard.

Season the chicken, then brown 3–4 pieces at a time in the frying pan. Transfer them to a very large saucepan. When you have finished browning all the chicken, discard the oil.

Add the potatoes, carrots, olives and bay leaf to the saucepan, including the brine used to preserve the olives and any chicken bones. These will add to the flavour of the stock as the chicken cooks. Add both the paprikas to the saucepan and stir well.

Top up the saucepan with enough water to cover the chicken and vegetables and bring to the boil. Reduce the heat and simmer for one hour or until tender.

After about 45 minutes, remove several chunks of potato from the saucepan and place in a small bowl. Mash the potato with a fork, return it to the saucepan and stir. It will thicken the cooking liquid a little. Season the chicken and vegetables if required, and serve the chicken in large bowls with a sprinkling of parsley or coriander.

Fried rice with sesame beef and vegetables

A stir-fry is a useful dish to make if you have a sensitive gut, because you can tailor the ingredients to suit you. It can also be a healthy, nutritionally balanced dish because you can add starchy carbohydrate, a mixture of vegetables and a portion of meat, fish or tofu.

This is one of the fastest recipes in the book. It has lovely vibrant colours and fabulous flavours, but be sure to use a very good-quality, tender cut of steak.

SERVES 4
Hands-on time 10 minutes
Cooking time 15 minutes

2 tbsp rapeseed or other light-flavoured cooking oil
1 garlic clove, sliced
200 g/7 oz sirloin (strip loin) steak, trimmed and sliced into 1 cm/½ in strips
2 tbsp dark soy sauce, plus more to serve (optional)
walnut-sized piece of root ginger, peeled and grated
1 tbsp sesame seeds
250 g/9 oz/1⅓ cups long-grain rice
¼ tsp salt
100 g/4 oz/⅔ cup green beans, cut into 5 cm/2 in lengths
1 red (bell) pepper, deseeded and cut into strips
8 water chestnuts, sliced
1 tbsp chopped chives
1 tbsp chopped coriander (cilantro) leaves

Warm the oil in a wok and cook the garlic until it is just beginning to brown. Discard the garlic and leave the oil to cool a little. Place the strips of steak in a bowl with 1 tbsp of the garlic-infused oil, the soy sauce, ginger and sesame seeds. Mix together and leave to marinate for 10 minutes.

Pour the rice into a measuring jug and make a note of its volume. Place the rice in a saucepan with twice its volume of water and the salt. Bring to the boil, then reduce to a gentle simmer and place a lid on the saucepan. Simmer very gently for 12 minutes. Halfway through the cooking, quickly lift the lid and add the green beans so they can steam. Replace the lid and continue cooking.

Heat the remaining oil in the wok and stir-fry the red pepper until soft. Add the beef and fry briskly for 2 minutes, followed by the cooked rice and green beans. Toss the contents of the wok together, scraping up any residue on the base. Add the water chestnuts and any leftover marinade, and stir-fry for a further 2 minutes. Scatter the herbs into the wok and serve with soy sauce, if required.

TRY THIS:
• *Replace the steak with pork or prawns, or a combination of two of these ingredients.*
• *Add more vegetables, tofu, peanuts or sesame seeds for vegetarians.*

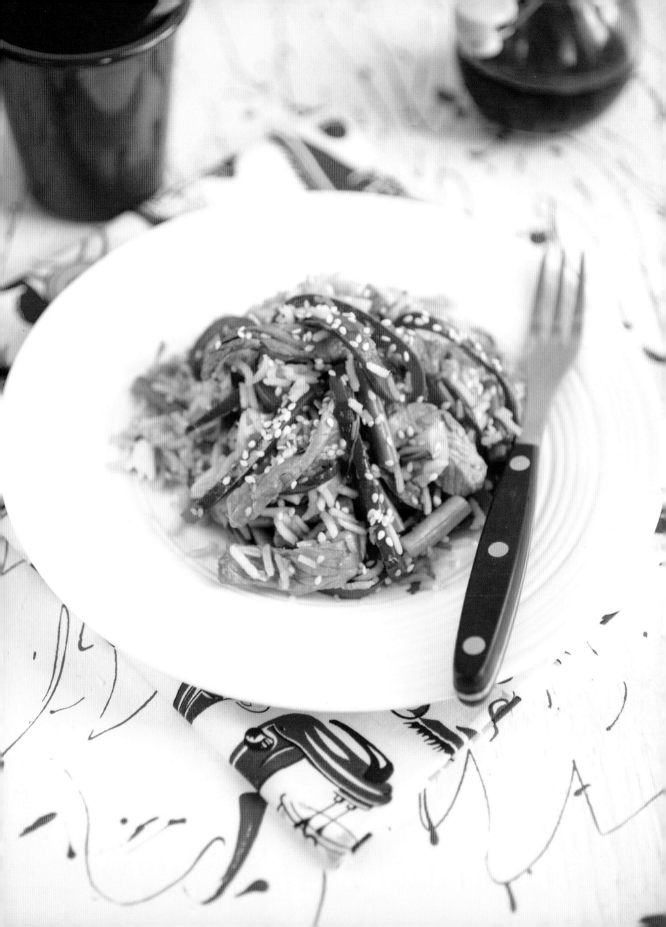

Chicken noodle pho

Thread-thin rice noodles are the thing to eat if you want some energy but you are feeling a little delicate. Pho is a fragrant, nutritious soup, South-East Asian street food at its best, containing a small amount of fish or meat with a variety of vegetables depending on the season. In this recipe, we have chosen vegetables that are low in FODMAPs and added just a little marinated chicken. Pho usually contains chillies, but we left them out as they can trigger symptoms in some people. Make your own stock or use just a small amount of a ready-made stock that you trust not to upset you. If in doubt, use water instead and flavour your pho with just a little soy sauce, fish sauce and lime juice.

SERVES 4
Hands-on time 10 minutes
Cooking time 10 minutes

200 g/8 oz/1¼ cups thread-thin
    rice noodles
200 g/7 oz/1¼ cups chicken, cut
    into thin strips
1 tbsp grated root ginger
2 cm/1 in length of lemongrass
    stalk, finely chopped
2 tbsp vegetable oil, such as
    rapeseed oil
sea salt and ground black pepper
200 g/7 oz/about 2 cups mixed
    vegetables such as pak choi,
    carrots, bean sprouts
green leaves of 4 spring onions
    (scallions), finely sliced
1 red (bell) pepper, deseeded
    and finely sliced
800 ml/1¼ pints/3 cups home-
    made Vegetable stock (p.44)
1 tbsp fish sauce, or to taste
juice of 1 lime, or to taste
1 tbsp soy sauce, or to taste
2 tbsp chopped fragrant herbs,
    such as coriander (cilantro),
    mint and chives

Place the noodles in a bowl and cover with boiling water. Leave to soak for 5 minutes, then drain. Set aside.

Slice the chicken and place it in a small bowl with the ginger, lemongrass and 1 tbsp of the oil. Season and mix well.

Prepare the vegetables: chop the carrots into matchstick-like strips and slice the pak choi.

Heat the remaining oil in a wok and gently sweat the spring onion tops and pepper until soft. Add the marinated chicken, with its marinade, and stir-fry briskly until the chicken begins to colour. Pour in the stock, fish sauce and lime juice, and bring it to a simmer.

Add the vegetables and cook for about 8 minutes until they are soft but retain some 'bite'.

When there are 4 minutes before serving, add the noodles to the wok. Taste the pho and season with soy sauce, fish sauce and a little more lime juice if required. Serve in bowls scattered with fragrant herbs.

TRY THIS:
• *Make this suitable for vegetarians by substituting the chicken with tofu.*
• *Cook the chicken on a griddle to create charred lines and develop its flavour.*

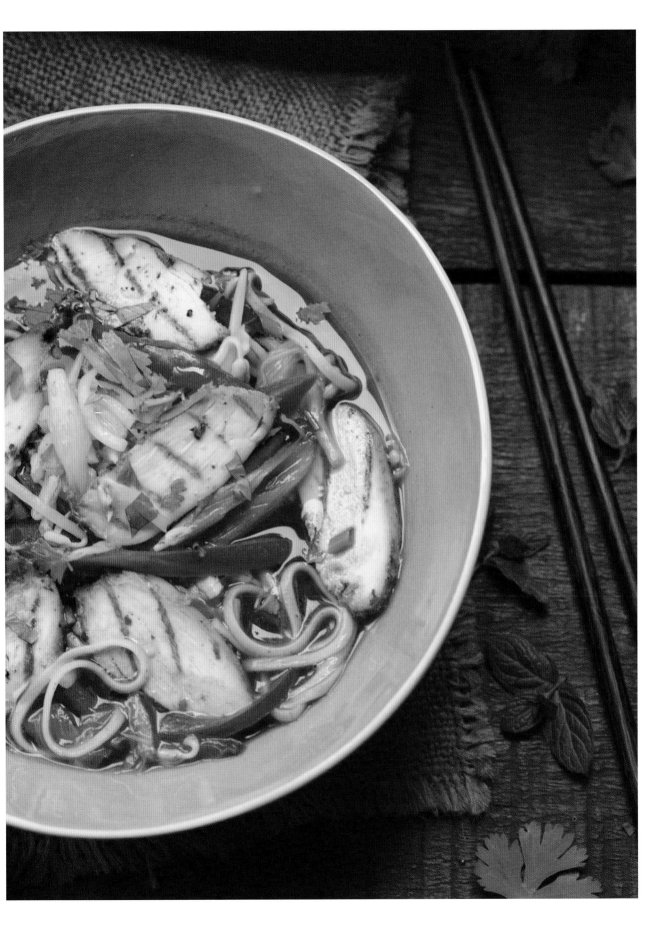

Aromatic tray-baked chicken

A well-cooked chicken dish can easily be made with ingredients that do not upset the gut.

We have served this for both a special occasion and an everyday meal because it is colourful and tasty. It can also be left in the oven, on a reduced heat, for a little longer than the stated cooking time if your schedule does not go quite according to plan.

This could be served with a dish of simply cooked polenta or roasted potato wedges.

SERVES 4
Hands-on time 15 minutes
Cooking time 1 hour

16 cherry tomatoes
1 red (bell) pepper, deseeded
  and thinly sliced
8 skinless, boneless free-range
  chicken thighs
leaves from 4 sprigs of rosemary
1 tsp sweet paprika
2 tbsp Garlic-infused oil (see
  p.36)
2 tbsp balsamic vinegar
sea salt and freshly ground
  black pepper
1 fennel bulb, trimmed and
  quartered lengthways
225 g/8 oz/1½ cups green beans
leaves from a small bunch of basil

Preheat the oven to 180°C/350°F/gas 4.

Place the tomatoes in a large roasting tray roughly 30 x 25 cm (12 x 10 in), with the pepper, chicken and rosemary.

Sprinkle the paprika, garlic oil, balsamic vinegar and a good pinch of salt and pepper over the chicken. Toss all the ingredients together and then spread the chicken thighs across the tray.

Place in the oven for 1 hour.

About halfway through the cooking time, steam the fennel and green beans for 5 minutes, or until both are tender, then drain well.

Remove the chicken and vegetables from the oven, add the fennel and baste it with the cooking juices from the chicken.

5 minutes before you are due to serve the chicken, add the steamed green beans and baste them with a little of the cooking juices. Return the roasting tray to the oven.

Serve with torn basil leaves and Oven-baked potatoes with rosemary and garlic oil (p.141) or Polenta (p.38).

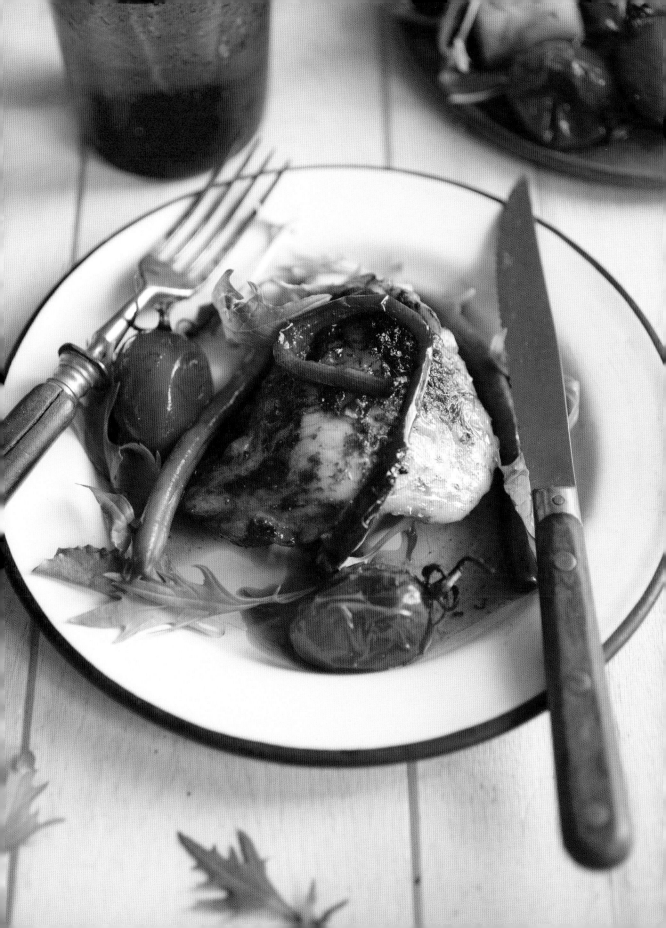

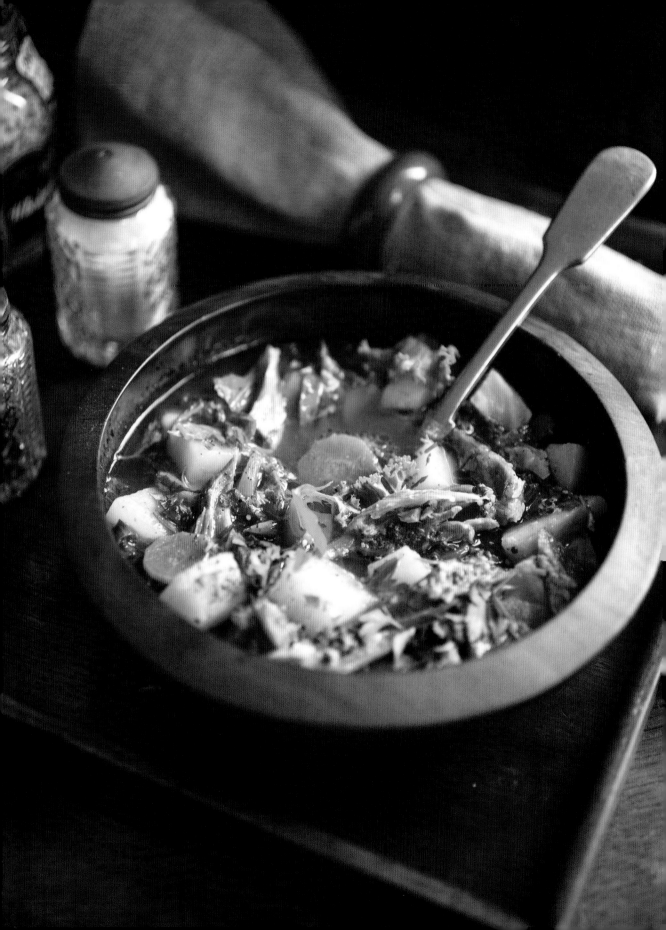

Shredded ham hock with kale

Kale is one green vegetable most people with a sensitive gut can eat. Its dark-green, frilly leaves are a rich source of beta carotene, vitamin C, vitamin K, folic acid, fibre and potassium, which all help to keep us healthy. Kale teams up well with a slow-cooked ham hock to produce a flavoursome stock. If you have extra stock from cooking the ham, you can use it in soups or freeze it for use later.

Ham is also delicious with a few canned lentils, which can be tolerated by most people as the fermentable carbohydrates leach out of them during the canning process. If you are not keen on lentils, just leave them out. This is ideal to cook at the weekend to be eaten during the week.

SERVES 4
Hands-on time 15 minutes
Cooking time 1¾ hours

TO COOK THE HOCK
1 small ham hock,
   weighing 860 g/2 lb
1 green leek leaf, roughly
   chopped
1 carrot, roughly chopped
1 celery stalk
1 bay leaf

TO MAKE THE DISH
2 tbsp olive oil
50 g/2 oz/½ cup tender green
   leek leaves, finely chopped
1 carrot, sliced
150 g/5 oz/1 cup celeriac, peeled
   and diced
2 small potatoes, peeled, cut into
   2 cm/1 in dice
100 g/3½ oz/½ cup canned
   lentils, drained and rinsed
large handful of kale, stalks
   removed, shredded
sea salt and ground black pepper
1 tbsp chopped parsley leaves

Place the ham hock in a large saucepan with the leek, carrot, celery and bay. Cover with water. Bring to the boil and simmer gently for 1½ hours, or longer if you have the time. Remove the saucepan from the heat and allow it to cool a little before lifting the ham hock from the stock. When the hock is cool enough to handle, shred the meat and discard the fat and skin. Strain the cooking liquid and set aside.

Add the olive oil to a large pan and add the leek leaves, carrot and celeriac and potatoes, and cook gently for 10 minutes or until the vegetables are soft. Add 600 ml/1 pint/2½ cups of cooking liquid from the ham hock and the lentils.

Add the kale and ham, and simmer for 5 minutes. Season the dish and serve in bowls scattered with parsley. Make sure there's a pot of mustard on the table.

Meatballs in herby tomato sauce

This recipe needs a few breadcrumbs to bind the meatballs. Although bread made from wheat contains fructans, most people can tolerate a slice (25 g/1 oz). Breadcrumbs made from gluten-free bread can be substituted if preferred (for home-made Gluten-free bread, see p.51).

This fabulous supper dish can be made ahead of time and frozen. It will keep for up to three months in a freezer.

These would be great served with Courgetti (see p.82), buckwheat noodles, pasta or polenta (see p.38).

SERVES 4
Hands-on time 15 minutes
Cooking time 30 minutes,
    plus 30 minutes chilling

leaves from 4 sprigs of rosemary,
    finely chopped
2 heaped tsp Dijon mustard
300 g/10½ oz/1⅓ cups quality
    lean minced (ground) beef
1 heaped tbsp dried oregano
2 slices of white bread, made into
    breadcrumbs
1 egg, lightly beaten
sea salt and freshly ground
    black pepper
1 quantity Basic tomato sauce
    (see p.46)
olive oil
50 g/2 oz/½ cup Parmesan
    cheese, finely grated
handful of basil leaves

Place the rosemary, mustard, minced beef, oregano and breadcrumbs in a bowl and add the egg and a pinch of salt and pepper. Mix well, divide into 16 and roll into tight balls with your hands. Place on a plate, cover and put in the fridge to become firm for at least 30 minutes, or while you make the tomato sauce (see p.46).

Heat a large frying pan and cover the base with olive oil. Add the meatballs and cook for 8–10 minutes, until beginning to brown. Open one of the meatballs up to check that it is cooked; it should not be pink in the middle.

Add the meatballs to the tomato sauce and pour in a little water if you need to so that the meatballs are half-submerged. Bring to the boil, then reduce the heat and simmer for 10 minutes. Serve with grated Parmesan and torn basil leaves.

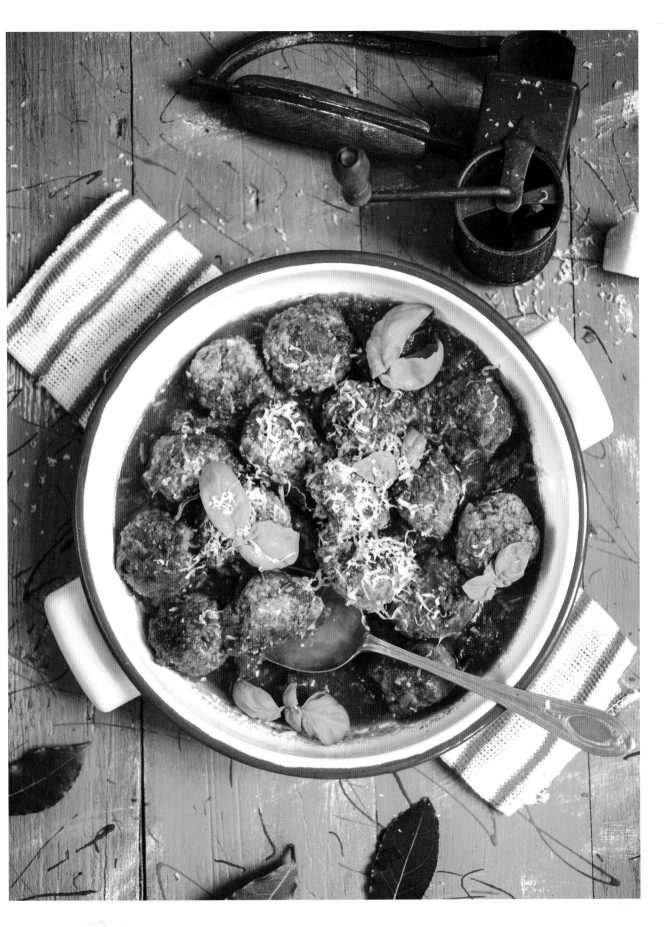

Ragù Bolognese

Many years ago, Joan spent six weeks in Bologna in Italy and learned how to make a classic Bolognese ragù. The cook who taught her showed her how to develop the rich, deep flavours by cooking it slowly and seasoning not only with garlic but herbs, a little bacon and even a chicken liver if available.

In Italy, less is more when it comes to serving a sauce with pasta. The sauce, rich, thick and full of flavour, should coat the pasta rather than drown it.

Joan has adapted her Bolognese sauce for people with a sensitive gut, omitting garlic and onions. It tastes good with polenta, spaghetti or in lasagne for a lovely satisfying meal.

SERVES 4

Hands-on time 10 minutes

Cooking time 1 hour

2 tbsp olive oil

2 garlic cloves, sliced

green leaves from 4 young leeks, finely sliced

½ celery stalk, finely chopped

500 g/1 lb/2 cups lean minced (ground) beef

100 g/4 oz/1 cup carrots, peeled and grated

1 glass (150 ml/5 fl oz/⅔ cup) red wine

400 g/14 oz can of plum tomatoes

1 bay leaf

½ tsp dried oregano

1 tbsp tomato purée (paste)

sea salt and freshly ground black pepper

50 g/2 oz/½ cup Parmesan cheese, finely grated (optional)

torn basil leaves (optional)

Gently heat the oil in a large saucepan and add the garlic. Cook gently until it just begins to brown. Remove the garlic from the pan and discard.

Add the leek leaves and celery to the garlic-flavoured oil and sweat gently until soft. Sear the mince until it is brown and then stir in the grated carrots.

Increase the heat under the saucepan, pour in the red wine and allow it to evaporate. Add the tomatoes and break them up a little bit with a wooden spoon. Add 200 ml/7 fl oz/¾ cup of water, the bay leaf, oregano and tomato purée to the sauce and season well.

Cover the saucepan and allow to cook gently for 40 minutes. Remove the lid and cook the sauce for another few minutes to thicken it if necessary.

Serve the sauce with gluten-free pasta, buckwheat noodles or Courgetti (see p.82). Grated Parmesan cheese and a few leaves of torn basil strewn over the sauce is always tasty.

Home-made pork and rosemary sausages with lentils

Everyone loves a sausage, but most ready-made sausages contain wheat and other cereals that may upset you. This recipe is tailored to the sensitive gut.

It takes its inspiration from a classic Umbrian lentil and sausage stew, using canned lentils to reduce the content of galacto-oligosaccharides (GOS). But these sausages would be equally at home on a plate of mashed potatoes, if you fancy something a little more British.

SERVES 4
Hands-on time 15 minutes
Cooking time 15 minutes

FOR THE SAUSAGES
500 g/1 lb 2 oz/2½ cups minced
   (ground) pork
2 tbsp dry white wine
1 tsp chopped rosemary leaves
sea salt and freshly ground
   black pepper

FOR THE DISH
3 tbsp olive oil
1 carrot, finely chopped
150 g/5 oz/¾ cup potatoes,
   chopped into 1 cm/½ in cubes
1 celery stalk, finely chopped
10 cherry tomatoes
200 g/7 oz/1 cup canned green
   lentils, drained
1 tsp Garlic-infused oil (see p.36)

Mix together the pork, wine and rosemary, and season well. Divide the mixture into 8 and roll each into a sausage 12 cm/5 in long and 3 cm/1½ in across. Wrap each tightly in foil and twist the ends as you would a sweet.

Bring a large pan of water to the boil. Poach the sausages in the boiling water for 3 minutes. Leave to cool, then remove the foil. (The poaching ensures the sausages hold together.)

Pour 2 tbsp of the oil into a frying pan and cook the sausages until golden on all sides.

Place the remaining 1 tbsp of oil in a separate pan and sweat the carrot, potatoes and celery. Pour enough water into the pan to cover the vegetables and add the cherry tomatoes. Cover the saucepan and continue to cook for 5 minutes or until the vegetables are soft. Add the lentils and allow them to heat through. Lay the browned sausages on top and cook gently for another 5 minutes, making sure everything is piping hot. Drizzle the garlic oil over before serving.

Shepherd's pie with buttered swede

The trick here is to add a little soy sauce to the filling. It really enhances the flavour and adds a deep brown colour. It is important not to add too much fat to mashed potatoes, as fat may trigger symptoms in a sensitive gut. Instead, use lactose-free milk. You can freeze this in a suitable container for up to three months. Thaw it thoroughly and cook at 200°C/325°F/gas 6 for 25 minutes.

SERVES 4
Hands-on time 20 minutes
Cooking time 1 hour

FOR THE FILLING
2 tbsp oil
1 tbsp finely chopped green
   leaves of leek
500 g/1 lb/2 cups lean minced
   (ground) beef
100 g/4 oz/1 cup carrot, chopped
2 tbsp cornflour (cornstarch)
1 bay leaf
1 tbsp dark soy sauce
1 tbsp tomato purée (paste)
2 tsp Dijon mustard
sea salt and ground black pepper

FOR THE TOPPING
500 g/1 lb/2½ cups potatoes,
   peeled and cut into chunks
4 tbsp lactose-free milk
1 tbsp olive oil
1 tbsp finely chopped chives,
   parsley or sage leaves

FOR THE SWEDE
400 g/7 oz/2 cups swede (yellow
   turnip), peeled, chopped into
   3 cm/1½ in chunks
15 g/½ oz/1 tbsp unsalted butter
1 tbsp chopped parsley

Gently heat the oil in a large non-stick saucepan and add the leek leaves. Sweat gently until soft.

Sear the mince in the same pan until it is brown and add the carrots. Stir in the cornflour and cook for 2 minutes.

Pour 500 ml/18 fl oz/2 cups of water into the saucepan and add the bay leaf, soy sauce, tomato purée and Dijon mustard. Season well. Give the mince a good stir, increase the heat and bring it to a simmer. Cover the saucepan, reduce the heat and cook gently for 40 minutes.

Remove the lid from the pan and cook the meat sauce for another few minutes to allow some of the liquid to evaporate so that the filling is moist but not too sloppy.

Cook the potatoes in plenty of boiling, salted water for 12–15 minutes or until soft. Drain and allow them to cool slightly before mashing them. Add enough milk to form a stiff paste and stir in a little olive oil.

Place the filling in an ovenproof dish and spread the mashed potato over the top. Place under a hot grill to brown for about 10 minutes.

Meanwhile, boil the swede in a saucepan of salted water for about 10 minutes or until tender. Drain and serve with the melted butter and parsley, seasoning well.

Serve the shepherd's pie scattered with chopped, fresh herbs.

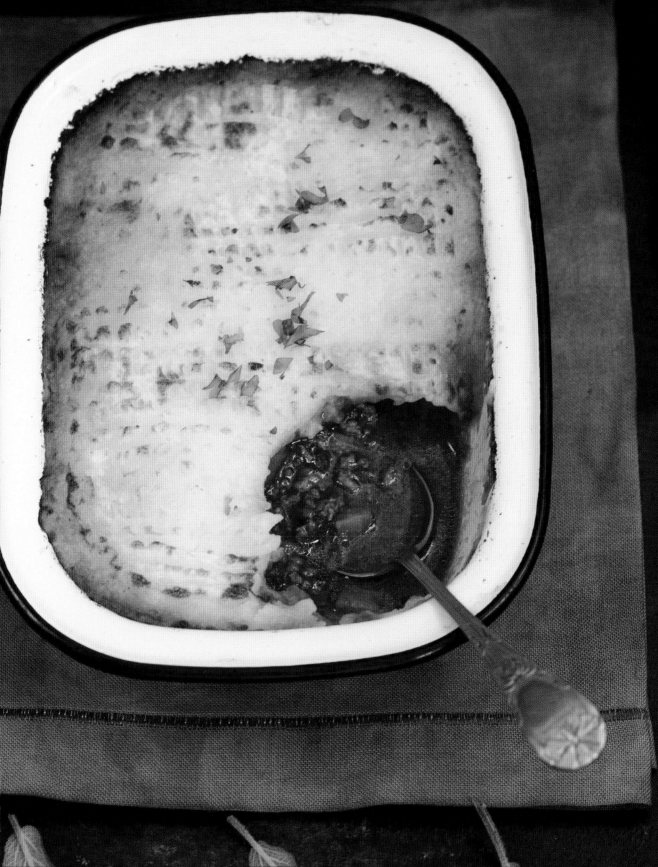

Lamb shanks with red wine, root vegetables and woody herbs

This dish is so quick to prepare but slow to cook; the pot is parked in the oven for 1½ hours while you do something else. During this time, the flavours of the rosemary and bay mingle with the red wine and the juices from the cooking meat and vegetables. The result is glorious. Perhaps the only other ingredient you might like with it is some steamed kale.

SERVES 4
Hands-on time 10 minutes
Cooking time 1½ hours

500 g/1 lb/2 cups parsnips,
    peeled and cut into chunks
500 g/1 lb/2 cups carrots, peeled
    and cut into chunks
2 lamb shanks
3 sprigs of rosemary
1 bay leaf
sea salt and freshly ground
    black pepper
500 ml/18 fl oz/2 cups red wine

Preheat the oven to 180°C/350°F/gas 4.

Place the vegetables in the base of a large casserole dish and lay the lamb shanks on top, followed by the herbs. Season the lamb with salt and pepper. Pour the wine over and add 300 ml/10 fl oz/1¼ cups of water, so the lamb is half-submerged. Season well.

Cover the dish with a lid and cook in the oven for 1½ hours, by which time the lamb should be succulent and tender. Just before serving, remove the lamb and place on a warmed plate to rest for a few minutes before carving the meat from the bones. Cover the meat with foil to keep warm.

Roughly mash the parsnips and carrots into the gravy. Serve the mashed vegetables and gravy topped with slices of meat.

TRY THIS:
• *Use water instead of wine. Just add enough water to come halfway up the lamb and cook as above.*
• *2 anchovies can be added to the sauce to make a savoury gravy.*
• *Add juniper berries for an interesting flavour.*

Warm potato and pastrami salad with dill and mustard dressing

This combination is wonderful and very sustaining. Although mustard tastes hot, it does not contain capsaicin, the component in chillies that can irritate the intestine. A few gherkins (1 tbsp) will be tolerated by most people with a sensitive gut. The salad ingredients and herbs are all very soothing.

SERVES 4
Hands-on time 15 minutes
Cooking time 15 minutes

500 g/1 lb small new potatoes,
    scrubbed
1 head of crisp lettuce, leaves
    separated and rinsed
2 tomatoes, sliced
200 g/7 oz pastrami, cut into
    strips
8 gherkins, sliced
2 tbsp finely chopped dill
1 tbsp finely chopped chives

FOR THE DRESSING
1 tbsp wholegrain mustard
½ tsp light brown sugar
1 tbsp white wine vinegar
3 tbsp good-quality fruity olive oil
sea salt and freshly ground
    black pepper

Place the potatoes in a saucepan of boiling water and cook for 10–15 minutes until tender. Drain, return them to the saucepan and cover to keep warm.

Make the dressing by mixing the mustard, sugar, vinegar and olive oil in a jar and shake well. Season with salt and pepper.

Quickly tear the lettuce into small pieces and arrange in a bowl. Lay the potatoes, tomatoes, pastrami and gherkins on the lettuce. Scatter over the dill and chives and serve.

VEGETARIAN

We have created a range of interesting vegetarian dishes which use a whole gamut of ingredients that will help you to eat a healthy vegetarian diet. Although there are a lot of vegetables and fruits that contain substantial amounts of poorly absorbed fermentable sugars, there are more that don't, and they are great to include in vegetarian dishes.

Cheese is a really useful ingredient in vegetarian dishes and is rich in calcium and other important nutrients. Hard cheeses are low in lactose sugar, but may contain appreciable amounts of fat, so it is best to use them judiciously.

Roasted veg and goat's cheese muffins

These can be eaten for breakfast, a light meal or a snack. They contain a mixture of vegetables bound together with a cheesy egg mixture, rather like a frittata, but do not contain flour. The combination of vegetables can be chosen from our list of low-FODMAPs foods (see p.25). It is quite good to include vegetables that are suitable for roasting, such as parsnips and peppers, then mix them with shredded leaf vegetables such as kale or spinach. You just need enough vegetables to cover two baking trays. This will give you enough to fill the muffin tins.

MAKES 12 MUFFINS/SERVES 6
Hands-on time 10 minutes
Cooking time 35 minutes

420 g/15 oz/3 cups sweet potato
1 red (bell) pepper
1 courgette (zucchini)
1 parsnip
1–2 tbsp olive oil
sea salt and ground black pepper
8 eggs
75 g/3 oz/⅓ cup goat's cheese,
    cut into small pieces
basil leaves

Preheat the oven to 175°C/350°F/gas 4. Cut all the vegetables into 1 cm/½ in cubes. Place the vegetables on a baking tray and drizzle with the oil. Sprinkle with salt and pepper, and toss well to ensure they are coated with oil. Roast for 15–20 minutes or until tender.

Meanwhile, whisk the eggs and season with salt and pepper.

Line the muffin tins with muffin cases, or cut 12 x 12 cm/5 in squares of non-stick baking paper and scrunch them into the wells in the muffin tin.

Divide the roasted vegetables and goat's cheese between the muffin cases. Pour the egg mixture over and bake in the oven for 15 minutes or until just set and golden brown.

Sprinkle with a few torn basil leaves to serve.

Aubergine with tahini and pickled radishes

Aubergine (eggplant) is an exotic, mysterious, plump vegetable with beautiful deep-purple skin and is the mainstay of many Mediterranean and Middle Eastern dishes. A small portion of aubergine is fine to eat if you have a sensitive gut, but do not fry it in too much oil, because this vegetable acts like a sponge and absorbs it all. Just wipe the cut surface of sliced aubergine with a little oil, then place on a baking tray or in a large covered non-stick frying pan. Cover the aubergine with foil, or a lid, for the first 10 minutes of cooking. That way the steam created inside the pan will soften the flesh of the aubergine without the need for more oil.

Using a small amount of yogurt in the tahini dressing should be quite acceptable for most people with a sensitive gut. Alternatively, you can crumble a little feta cheese over the aubergine.

SERVES 4

Hands-on time 10 minutes

Cooking time 30 minutes

FOR THE PICKLED RADISHES

10–15 radishes, washed and
thinly sliced into rings

250 ml/9 fl oz/1 cup white wine
vinegar

1 tbsp sugar

1 tsp fine cooking salt

FOR THE AUBERGINE

2 aubergines (eggplants), cut into
rings 1.5 cm/¾ in thick

2 tbsp fine cooking salt

2 tbsp olive oil

6 tbsp Greek yogurt

1 tbsp tahini

lemon juice, to taste

sea salt and freshly ground
black pepper

2 tbsp chopped coriander
(cilantro) leaves

It is a good idea to make the pickled radishes a couple of hours before cooking the aubergines. Slice the radishes thinly and place them in a jar. Combine the vinegar, sugar and salt in a small saucepan and heat gently until the sugar and salt have dissolved. Bring to the boil, remove from the heat, pour over the sliced radishes and leave for a couple of hours. The radishes will soften slightly and take on a beautiful pink tone.

Preheat the oven to 200°C/400°F/gas 6.

Place the aubergine rings in a colander resting on a plate and sprinkle with the salt. Leave for 15 minutes to allow the salt to draw some of the moisture from the flesh. When you see drops of liquid collecting on the plate, rinse the aubergines well and wipe dry.

Place the aubergines on a baking tray or in a large ovenproof frying pan with a lid. Drizzle some olive oil over the baking tray and wipe each slice of aubergine in the oil to ensure it is coated with a fine film. Cover and bake in the oven for 20 minutes or until they are soft and their surfaces gently caramelised, turning halfway through. If you master this, then you will be on your way to be a great cook of Middle Eastern food.

To make the dressing, place the yogurt in a bowl with the tahini and add lemon juice a little at a time, tasting as you go. Add a little water if you need to loosen the dressing. Mix well and season.

Arrange the aubergine on a serving plate, topping each round with 1 tsp of dressing and a slice of pickled radish. Finish with chopped coriander.

Aubergine, quinoa, feta and herbs

Quinoa is a small gluten-free grain that can grow in inhospitable climates. Traditionally, it was ground into flour and made into baked products. It has a higher protein content than rice and it contains other useful micronutrients, such as calcium.

Quinoa has the potential to help to alleviate malnutrition across the world because it can grow where other grains cannot. It has also taken centre stage in gourmet kitchens because it has an unusual nutty flavour and pretty appearance. The small white, red or black grains unfurl when cooked to produce a curly 'tail' and look so attractive.

Quinoa is a great ingredient to use instead of wheat-based couscous and pasta, and works well with Mediterranean dishes. It is low in FODMAPs and should be tolerated by most people with a sensitive gut.

SERVES 4
Hands-on time 10 minutes
Cooking time 30 minutes

2 aubergines (eggplants)
2 tbsp cooking salt
1 tbsp olive oil
250 g/5 oz/1 cup quinoa
  (use 3-colour if you can find it)
2 tbsp pine nuts
100 g/3 oz/½ cup cherry
  tomatoes, chopped
1 tbsp chopped chives
1 tbsp chopped parsley leaves
150 g/5 oz/1 cup feta cheese,
  crumbled
sea salt and freshly ground
  black pepper
1 tbsp chopped coriander
  (cilantro) leaves

Preheat the oven to 200°C/400°F/gas 6. Cut the aubergines lengthways into 1.5 cm-/⅔ in-thick strips and lay on a plate. Sprinkle with the salt and leave for 15 minutes. When drops of moisture appear on the cut surfaces of the aubergines, rinse well under cold water and pat dry.

Drizzle a little olive oil on a baking tray and wipe the cut surfaces of the aubergines with the oil before arranging the slices in rows. Cover with foil and place in the oven for 10 minutes. Remove the foil and continue to cook until tender for a further 10 minutes.

Meanwhile, pour the quinoa into a measuring jug and make a note of its volume. Place the quinoa in a pan with twice its volume of water and bring to the boil. Reduce the heat and simmer for 8 minutes or until just tender. Drain and place in a bowl with the pine nuts, tomatoes, chives, parsley and feta, then season well.

When the aubergine slices are soft and beginning to turn golden brown, remove them from the oven and spread 1 tbsp of the quinoa mixture on the top of each slice. Return to the oven and cook for a further 10 minutes. Serve hot with a sprinkling of coriander.

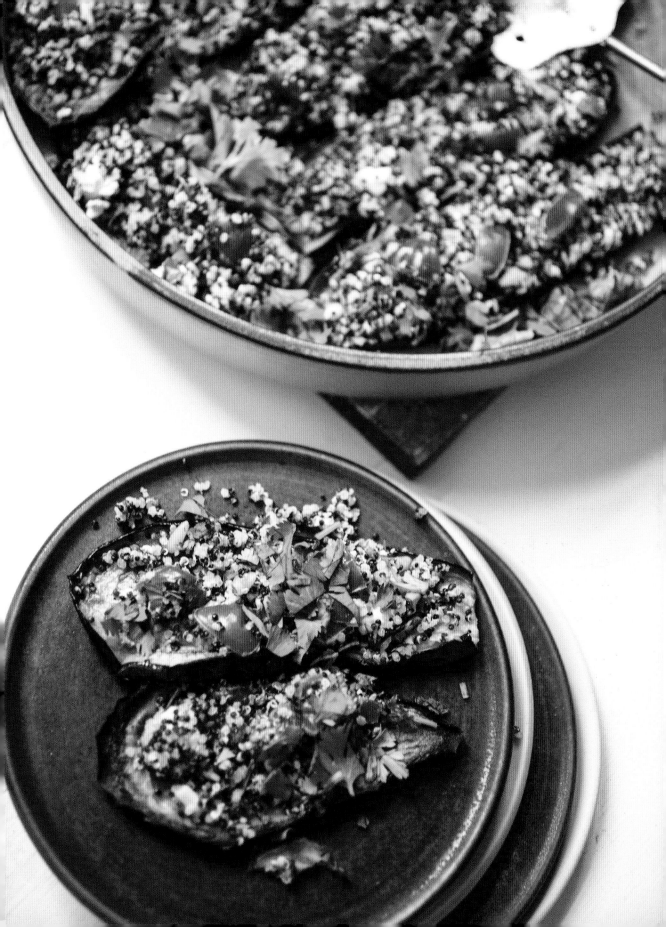

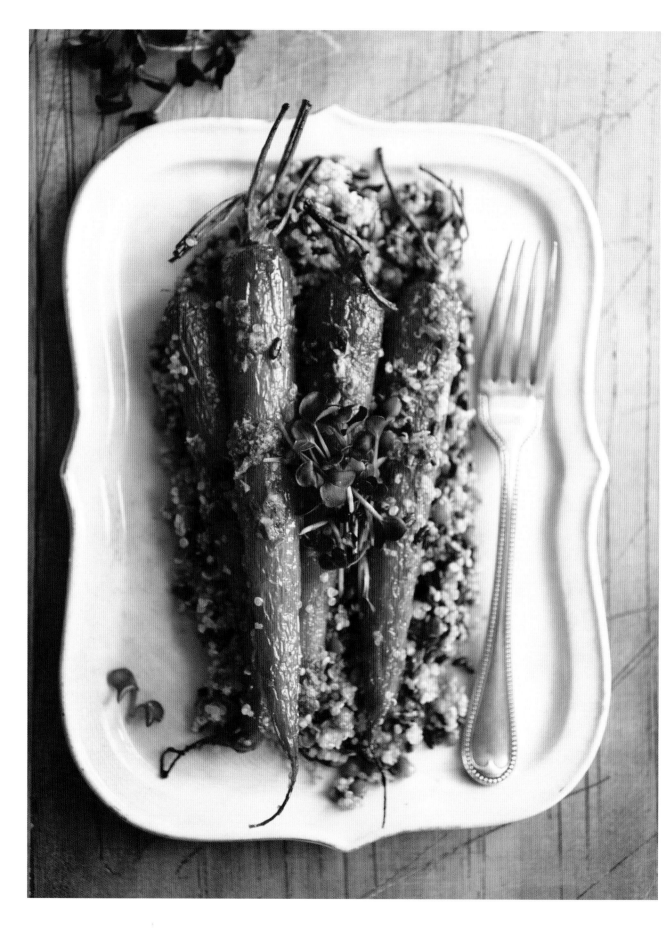

Roast carrots and mixed grains with rocket and feta dressing

This combination of deep-orange roasted carrots, green dressing and black rice not only looks beautiful, but tastes wonderful. Roasting develops the sweet flavour of carrots and gives them a soft-but-firm texture that goes well with the rice, rocket and feta. It can form a main course or a side dish.

If you are not happy eating black or brown rice, use white rice in this dish. The lentils add a nutty flavour and, if they have been canned rather than dried, are much better tolerated by a sensitive gut.

SERVES 4

Hands-on time 10 minutes

Cooking time 30 minutes

100 g/3½ oz/½ cup black rice
100 g/3½ oz/½ cup quinoa
100 g/3½ oz/½ cup canned
   lentils, drained and rinsed
8–10 young carrots, with their
   feathery leaves if possible
1 tbsp maple syrup
1 tbsp olive oil
1 tsp flaked sea salt

FOR THE DRESSING

50 g/2 oz/2 cups rocket (arugula)
120 ml/4 fl oz/½ cup olive oil
juice of ½ lemon, or to taste
100 g/3½ oz/⅔ cup feta cheese
sea salt and freshly ground
   black pepper

Preheat the oven to 200°C/400°F/gas 6.

Pour the black rice into a measuring jug and make a note of its volume. Place the rice in a saucepan with 3 times its volume of water. Bring to the boil, then reduce the heat and simmer for about 25 minutes or until cooked. Cook the quinoa in a separate pan with twice its volume of water for about 8 minutes, or until tender. Drain both grains, place in a bowl and stir in the lentils. Cover the bowl and keep warm.

Scrub the carrots and remove any feathery leaves but leave about 2 cm/ 1 in of the stem. Place in an ovenproof dish with the maple syrup, olive oil and salt. Roll the carrots around so they are well coated and bake for 20–30 minutes depending on their size. (Insert a sharp knife into the carrots to check they are soft in the middle.)

Liquidise the rocket, olive oil, lemon juice and feta to make the dressing. Taste and adjust the seasoning, adding a little more lemon juice if required.

Place the warm grains and lentils on a serving platter, top with the roasted carrots and pour over the dressing.

TRY THIS:
- *Use coriander (cilantro) instead of rocket to make the dressing.*
- *Use white, brown or red rice instead of black rice.*
- *Use Pesto (see p.48) instead of the rocket and feta dressing.*

Roasted vegetables with halloumi cheese and basil oil

A quick, healthy supper that can be eaten with quinoa, rice, potatoes or polenta. You can change the vegetables around a little to suit what you like and have available. A few green beans scattered over the finished dish would be nice. Halloumi is fine for most people to eat in small quantities (2 slices). The basil oil adds a bit of magic to this dish and any extra comes in useful for drizzling on sliced tomatoes and salads, but you could use Pesto instead (see p.48).

SERVES 4
Hands-on time 10 minutes
Cooking time 40 minutes

FOR THE ROASTED VEGETABLES
1 small fennel bulb, washed
1 medium courgette (zucchini), cut at an angle into 1 cm/½ in slices
1 red (bell) pepper, deseeded, cut into 8 pieces
280 g/10 oz/2 cups sweet potatoes, peeled, cut into 2 cm/1 in cubes
2 tbsp olive oil
sea salt and freshly ground black pepper
200 g/7 oz/8 slices halloumi cheese

FOR THE BASIL OIL
50 g/2 oz/2 cups basil leaves
75 ml/2 ½ fl oz/⅓ cup olive oil
sea salt and freshly ground black pepper
1½ tbsp lemon juice

Preheat the oven to 200°C/400°F/gas 6.

Remove any discoloured outer leaves from the fennel and trim the base. Set aside any fronds from the top. Cut the bulb into 8 pieces and plunge into a saucepan of boiling water to blanch for 5 minutes, or until just beginning to soften. Drain, refresh in cold water, then allow it to dry.

Put the fennel, courgette, pepper and sweet potato pieces in a roasting tin and toss with 1 tbsp of the olive oil to coat. Season with salt and mix well. Cook for 20 minutes. Open the oven door and move the vegetables around to ensure even cooking. Return the vegetables to the oven and cook for another 10 minutes or until soft and beginning to brown.

Slice the halloumi into 8 pieces, each about 1 cm/½ in thick, coat with the remaining oil and set aside.

Meanwhile, make the basil oil. Process the basil leaves in a food processor with the olive oil, a grind of black pepper and a pinch of sea salt. Gradually add the lemon juice to produce a vivid bright green sauce. Taste and adjust the seasoning.

To cook the halloumi, heat a heavy, ridged griddle pan on the hob. Place the halloumi on the griddle and cook until it is just beginning to melt and form dark ridges on its surface. Turn and cook until well browned on the other side.

Place the vegetables, any tender fronds from preparing the fennel, and the cheese in a serving bowl and serve with a drizzle of basil oil.

Fast black rice salad

This is lovely as a light meal or to team up with other dishes such as an omelette or tofu. If you do not have black rice, brown or red rice would be a good substitute. We love this because it is full of flavour and texture and very low in fat. The dressing is South-East Asian and tastes wonderful with rice.

SERVES 4

Hands-on time 10 minutes

Cooking time 25 minutes

FOR THE SALAD

100 g/3½ oz/½ cup black rice

½ red (bell) pepper

1 tbsp chopped green spring
   onion (scallion) leaves, or chives

8 cherry tomatoes, quartered

1 tsp grated root ginger

2 tbsp chopped coriander
   (cilantro) leaves

FOR THE DRESSING

2 tbsp soy sauce

2 tbsp fish sauce (optional)

finely grated zest and juice
   of 1 lime

¼ tsp caster (superfine) sugar

½ mild red chilli, deseeded, finely
   chopped (optional)

Place the rice in a saucepan with 500 ml/18 fl oz/2 cups of water. Bring to the boil, then reduce the heat and simmer for 25 minutes until tender. Take a little of the rice from the water with a fork and taste it: the grains should be chewy but not hard. Drain and place in a bowl.

Meanwhile, grill the pepper until the skin has charred. Allow to cool a little, then peel off the skin and remove any seeds. Cut the pepper into 1 cm/½ in strips and add to the cooked rice.

Add the spring onion leaves, tomatoes, ginger and coriander, and mix well.

Mix the soy sauce, fish sauce, lime zest and caster sugar in a small bowl. Gradually add half the lime juice, tasting as you mix and adding more lime juice as required. Add the chilli, if using. Mix the dressing and pour over the salad.

Shakshuka

This quick-to-make North African one-pot meal is packed with strong flavours and vivid colours. The ingredients can be varied. Some add shredded spinach or kale to the sauce, others preserved lemon or crumbled feta. Once you have tried the basic recipe, it is yours to play around with and make your own. Serve with some lightly sautéed potatoes.

SERVES 4
Hands-on time 10 minutes
Cooking time 20 minutes

2 tbsp olive oil
2 garlic cloves, sliced
1 red (bell) pepper, deseeded
    and cut into long thin strips
1 yellow (bell) pepper, deseeded
    and cut into long thin strips
1 tsp cumin seeds, ground
1 tsp sweet paprika
400 g/14 oz can of plum
    tomatoes
1 bay leaf
4 eggs
sea salt and freshly ground
    black pepper
handful of basil leaves, torn
1 tbsp chopped coriander
    (cilantro) leaves

Heat the olive oil in a frying pan that has a lid and add the garlic. Cook until it is just beginning to brown, then remove from the oil and discard. Add the peppers to the frying pan with the cumin and paprika. Cook gently until the peppers become soft. Place the tomatoes into the frying pan with the bay leaf and cook for about 10 minutes, or until the sauce thickens.

Make 4 indentations in the sauce and carefully crack the eggs into them. Season the eggs with a little salt and pepper. Cover the frying pan and cook for about 5 minutes or until the eggs are set. Serve the shakshuka strewn with the basil and coriander. This is good with sautéed potatoes.

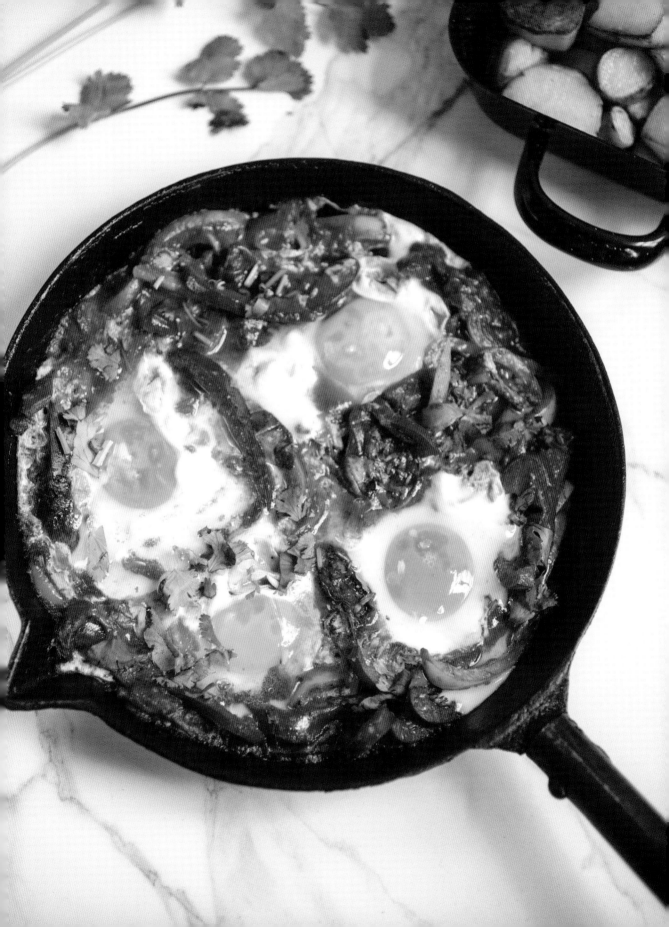

Sweet potato, courgette and herb frittata with pesto

This nutritious and satisfying one-pan meal is perfect and speedy to cook if you come home hungry after work. The vegetables can be varied depending what you have available and what suits you. You might, for example, substitute ordinary potatoes for sweet potatoes, or use a mix of both.

SERVES 4
Hands-on time 10 minutes
Cooking time 25 minutes

2 tbsp olive oil
300 g/10 oz/2 cups sweet
    potatoes, cut into
    2 cm/1 in cubes
2 courgettes (zucchini), pared into
    ribbons with a potato peeler
8 eggs
2 tbsp lactose-free milk
sea salt and freshly ground
    black pepper
4 tbsp finely grated Parmesan
    cheese
2 tbsp Pesto (see p.48)
small bunch of basil leaves, torn

Preheat the oven to 200°C/400°F/gas 6.

Heat a little olive oil in an ovenproof frying pan, about 20 cm/8 in across. Place in the sweet potatoes and cook gently for 10 minutes until soft. Add the courgette ribbons and continue to cook gently for another 5 minutes. Remove the vegetables from the frying pan and set aside.

In a bowl, whisk the eggs and milk together and season with a little salt and pepper.

Gently warm a non-stick frying pan and coat with a little olive oil. Pour the egg mixture into the pan and cook gently for about 7 minutes or until the frittata is just beginning to set. Carefully loosen the edges and bottom of the frittata to prevent it from burning.

Scatter the cooked vegetables evenly over the top of the frittata and continue to cook on the hob for another minute or so. Transfer to the oven and cook for about 5 minutes, or until it is just set in the middle and golden brown. Remove from the oven, cut into 4 and serve with the Parmesan, drizzled with the pesto and basil leaves.

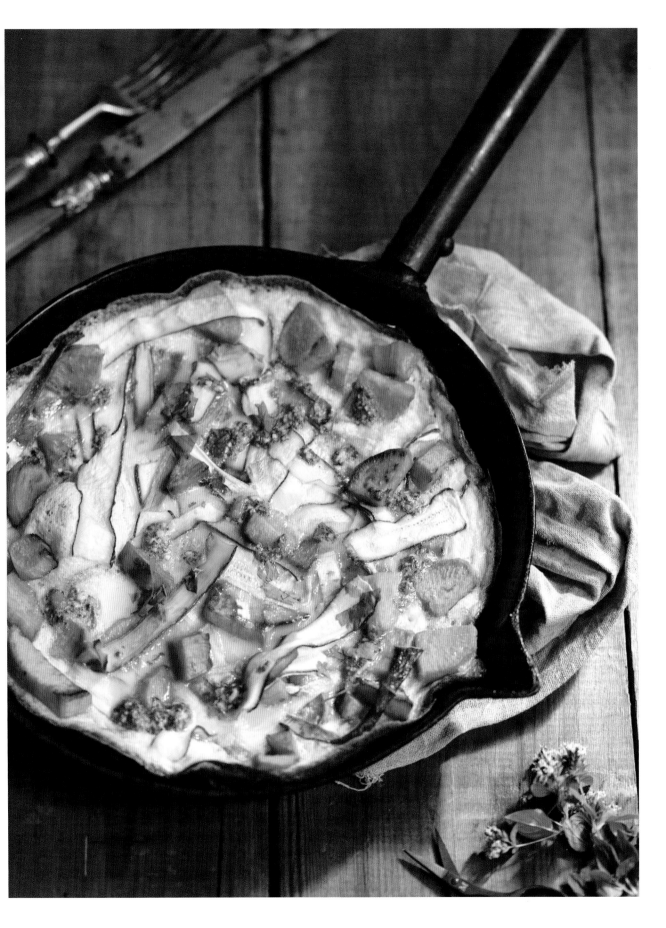

Buckwheat and spinach pancakes

These pancakes behave very nicely. They stay whole, are easy to turn over and look wonderful. Buckwheat is a great flour to use and can be tolerated by most people with a sensitive gut.

SERVES 4
Hands-on time 15 minutes
Cooking time 35 minutes

150 g/5 oz/1 cup buckwheat flour
2 eggs
330 ml/12 fl oz/1½ cups lactose-free milk
1 tsp melted coconut oil or unsalted butter
pinch of sea salt
2 handfuls of spinach
10 leaves of basil
1 tbsp chopped chives
a little grated nutmeg
2 tbsp olive oil
1 tsp pink peppercorns, crushed

FOR THE TOPPING
1 aubergine (eggplant), cubed
1 tbsp fine cooking salt
2 red (bell) peppers
1 tbsp olive oil
175 g/6 oz/⅔ cup canned chickpeas, drained and rinsed
1 tbsp black olives
1 tbsp chopped coriander (cilantro) leaves, extra to serve
sea salt and ground black pepper

FOR THE TAHINI CREAM
8 tbsp Greek yogurt
1 tbsp tahini
juice of 1 lemon, or to taste
½ tbsp Garlic-infused oil (p.36)

Place all the ingredients for the pancake batter, except the olive oil, in a large jug or bowl, stir in 150 ml/5 fl oz/⅔ cup of water and mix with a stick blender. Place in the fridge to settle while you prepare the topping.

Place the aubergine in a bowl, sprinkle with the salt and leave for 15 minutes or until droplets of water appear on the surfaces. Rinse the aubergine in running water to remove the salt. Place the aubergine in a covered pan with the olive oil to cook gently for about 15 minutes or until the flesh is soft and well cooked.

Hold the red peppers directly on the flame of a gas hob or on a grill and cook until the skin is scorched and black. Allow to cool before removing the blistered, black skin and the seeds. Cut the pepper into strips; do not be too fastidious about removing all the burnt skin as it adds a smoky flavour.

Add the chickpeas, black olives, peppers and coriander to the cooked aubergine. Season well and keep warm while you cook the pancakes.

Prepare the tahini cream by mixing all the ingredients together well. Taste and adjust the seasoning, adding more salt, pepper or lemon juice as required.

To cook the pancakes, heat a 20 cm/8 in frying pan over a medium heat. Add a little olive oil and, when it is hot, ladle about 100 ml/3 fl oz/⅓ cup of batter into the pan. Tilt the pan and swirl around until the batter is evenly distributed. Fry for about 2 minutes, until the pancakes are golden and can be turned over easily. Place on a baking tray in a warm oven while you cook the rest.

Place 2–3 spoonfuls of the red pepper topping in the centre of each pancake and spread around with a spoon. Place a dollop of tahini cream in the centre and sprinkle with pink peppercorns and a little more coriander before serving.

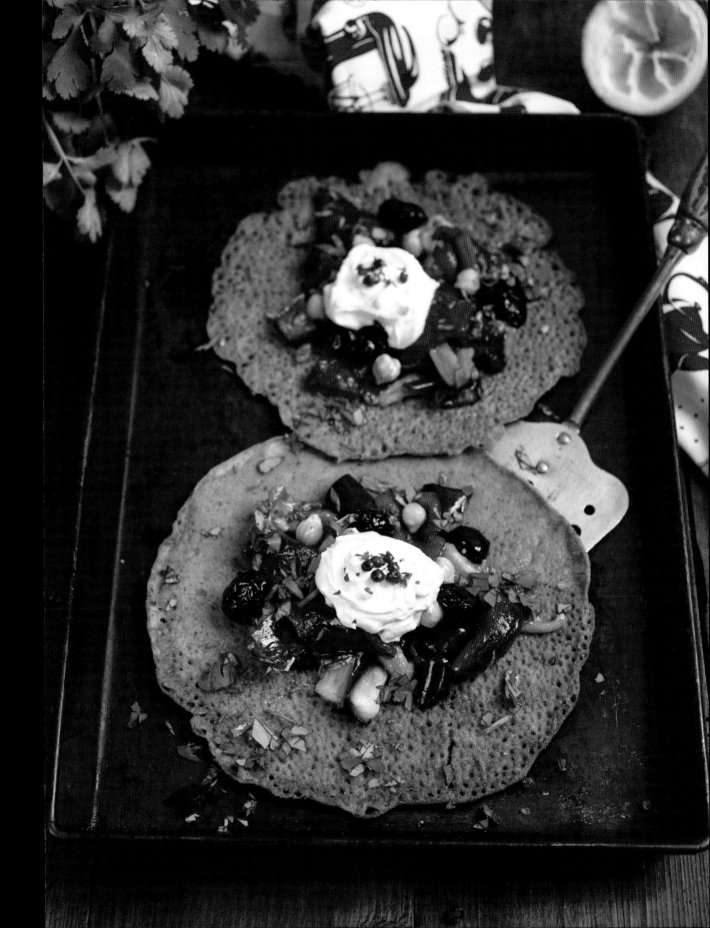

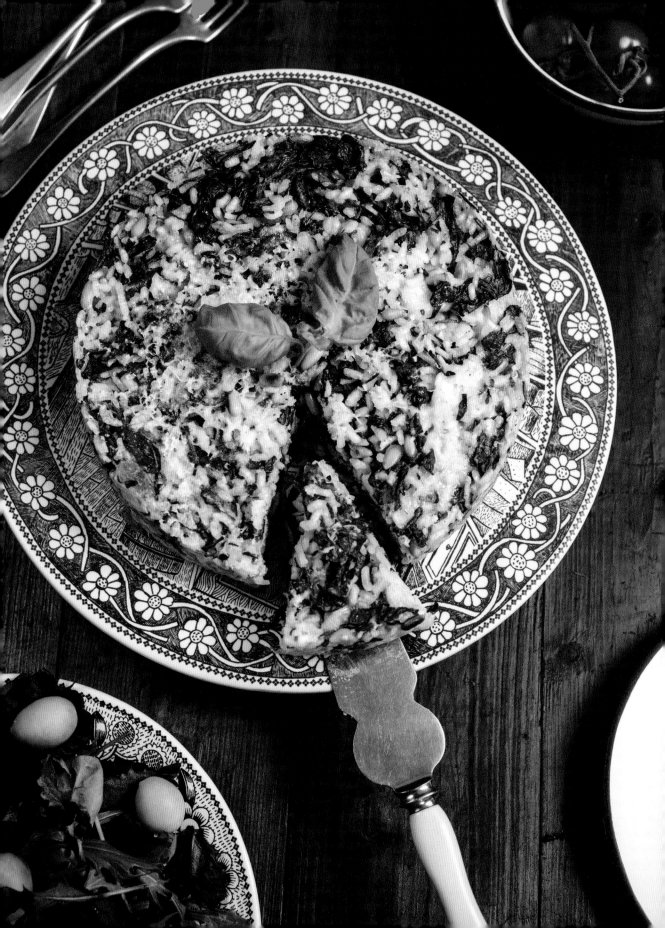

Spinach and rice torte

The gentle, complementary flavours of nutmeg and spinach make this a perfect dish to eat for lunch or a light evening meal. Rice is a good source of energy and is low in fermentable carbohydrates, so it is an ideal grain to use as a basis for meals if you have a sensitive gut. Serve this with a mixed salad or roasted vegetables. Any leftovers can be eaten the next day for lunch.

SERVES 4–6
Hands-on time 15 minutes
Cooking time 1 hour

500 g/1 lb/16 cups spinach,
   washed
250 g/9 oz/1¼ cups risotto rice
sea salt and freshly ground black
   pepper
10 g/½ oz/scant 1 tbsp unsalted
   butter
4 eggs, lightly beaten
1 tsp chopped sage leaves
1 tbsp chopped chives
50 g/1½ oz/⅓ cup pine nuts,
   toasted
freshly grated nutmeg
75 g/3 oz/¾ cup Parmesan
   cheese, freshly grated

Preheat the oven to 200°C/400°F/gas 6. Steam the spinach for 5 minutes, cool for a few minutes, then squeeze out as much moisture as possible. Roughly chop and set aside.

Tip the rice into a saucepan and add 600 ml/1 pint/2½ cups of water with a little salt. Bring to the boil, then reduce the heat to a simmer and cook, uncovered, for 10 minutes. By this time, the water should have been absorbed. Stir in the butter.

Place the eggs in a large bowl with the cooked spinach, sage, chives, toasted pine nuts, 2 generous pinches of sea salt, a generous grind of nutmeg and all but 1 tbsp of the Parmesan.

Mix the cooked rice into the spinach and egg mixture and stir well until combined. Spoon into a loose-based cake tin, measuring 20 cm/8 in across and 7 cm/3 in deep, lined with non-stick baking parchment, and sprinkle the remaining Parmesan over.

Cook for 25 minutes or until firm and beginning to brown. Remove from the oven and cool for 5 minutes.

Place a plate over the tin, invert the torte and peel off the parchment. Invert again on to a serving plate and serve.

Polenta pizza

This pizza is different. The middle of the polenta crust remains moist and adds a different dimension to eating a regular wheat dough base. The pizza is gluten-free and low in FODMAPs.

We have found making up batches of polenta quick and easy; sometimes the cooking instructions on the packets overestimate the time polenta takes to cook.

The great thing about making pizza is you can include the toppings that suit you and, if you are eating with other people, you can customise their pizza toppings, too.

MAKES 2 MEDIUM PIZZAS, ENOUGH FOR 4
Hands-on time 15 minutes
Cooking time 40 minutes

FOR THE TOPPING
2 red (bell) peppers, deseeded
   and cut into strips
2 courgettes (zucchini),
   shaved into ribbons with
   a potato peeler
2 tbsp Garlic-infused oil (see
   p.36), plus more for the trays
4 tomatoes, thinly sliced
1 tbsp capers, drained and rinsed
100 g/3 oz/⅔ cup olives, stoned
200 g/7 oz/2 cups mozzarella
handful of torn basil leaves

FOR THE BASES
160 g/6 oz quick-cook polenta
sea salt and freshly ground
   black pepper
30g/1 oz/2 tbsp unsalted butter
2 tsp finely chopped oregano
   leaves

Preheat the oven to 200°C/400°F/gas 6. Lay the peppers and courgettes on a baking tray and drizzle with the garlic oil. Roast for about 15 minutes or until soft, then set aside. Keep the oven on.

Place 1 litre/1¾ pints/1 quart of water in a saucepan and bring to the boil. Add the polenta in a thin stream and stir well. Continue to cook for 5 minutes, stirring continuously. It is cooked when it has formed a thick paste and leaves the sides of the pan. Season with salt and pepper, and stir in the butter and oregano.

Make 2 pizza bases by spreading the polenta on to 2 lightly oiled baking trays, making oval shapes about 25 cm/10 in long. Cook for 10 minutes to allow a skin to form. Remove from the oven.

Arrange the sliced tomatoes, peppers, courgettes and other topping ingredients over the bases and top with mozzarella (not the basil yet). Cook for 10–15 minutes or until the mozzarella bubbles. Remove from the oven, scatter with the basil and serve with a salad.

TRY THIS:
• Substitute feta cheese or goat's cheese for mozzarella.
• Add Parma ham for a meat version.

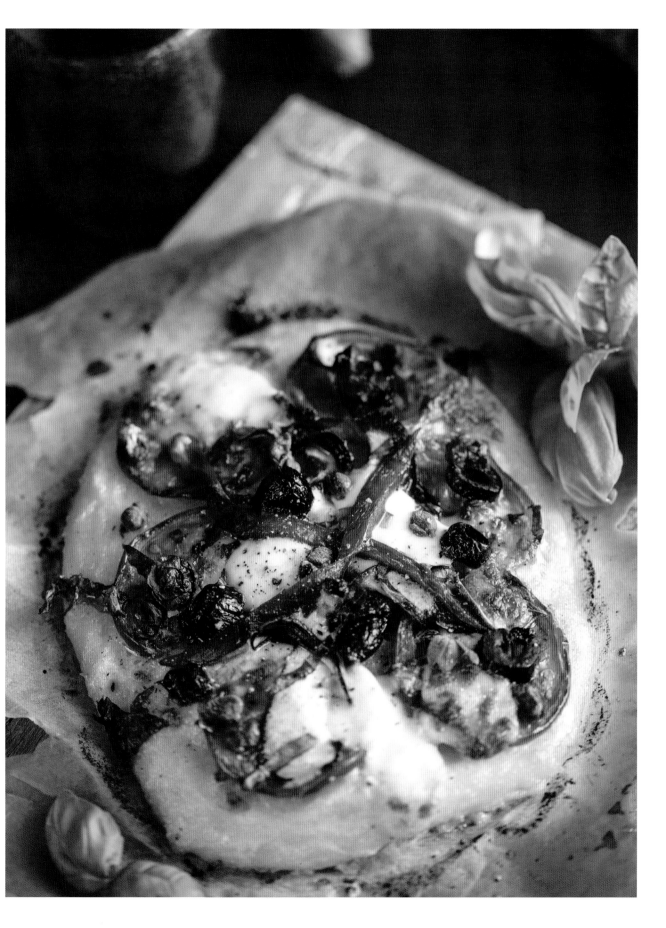

Spinach and Parmesan soufflé

This is a simple, quick recipe, somewhere between a soufflé and a frittata, which you can try out with different vegetables. The buckwheat flour and ground sunflower seeds add energy, essential fats and fibre to the mix, making it a substantial supper dish. Any leftovers can be eaten cold with a salad.

SERVES 4
Hands-on time 10 minutes
Cooking time 50 minutes

1 tbsp olive oil
½ tsp chives, snipped
    into ½ cm/¼ in lengths
180 g/6 oz/2½ cups shredded
    greens, such as chard,
    spinach or kale
½ tsp thyme leaves
1 tbsp finely chopped
    parsley leaves
6 eggs
500 ml/18 fl oz/2 cups lactose-
    free milk
60 g/2 oz/½ cup buckwheat flour
60 g/2 oz/⅓ cup sunflower seeds,
    ground
25 g/1 oz/¼ cup Parmesan
    cheese, grated,
    plus more to serve
sea salt and freshly ground
    black pepper
15 g/½ oz/1 tbsp unsalted butter
8 cherry tomatoes, halved

Preheat the oven to 200°C/400°F/gas 6.

Pour the oil into a non-stick frying pan and sweat the chives and shredded greens until soft. Remove from the heat, add the thyme and parsley, and mix well.

In a bowl whisk together the eggs and milk until frothy. Stir in the buckwheat flour, ground sunflower seeds and Parmesan. Fold in the cooked, shredded greens. Season with salt and pepper, and give the mixture a final stir.

Pour the egg and vegetable mixture into a generously buttered baking dish measuring 25 x 20 cm (10 x 8 in). Arrange the tomatoes on top and cook for about 45 minutes until golden brown. Remove from the oven and dust with Parmesan before serving.

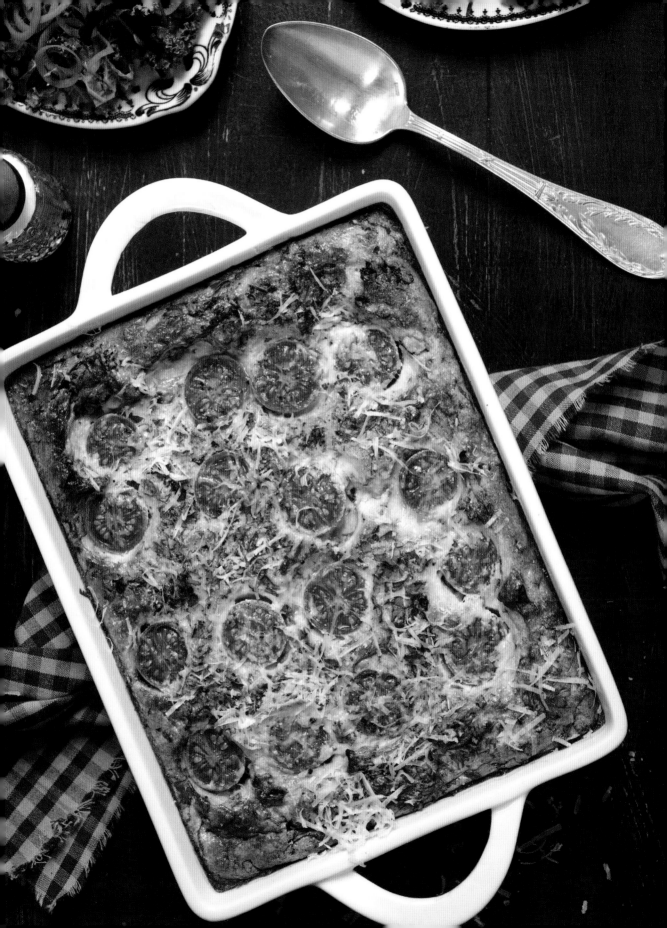

Courgetti with ginger, sunflower seeds and noodles

This is a very quick recipe which is ideal for when you are hungry and need something delicious on the table quickly. It has a wonderful balance of ingredients that are gentle on the gut and easily digested.

Courgetti can be made with a spiraliser or a julienne cutter. Or you can make ribbons of courgette with a potato peeler. Each of these methods produces lovely thin strips of courgette that stir-fry beautifully.

SERVES 4
Hands-on time 10 minutes
Cooking time 10 minutes

80 g/3 oz/½ cup vermicelli rice
     noodles
3 courgettes (zucchini)
3 tbsp rapeseed or olive oil
2 garlic cloves, sliced
1 tbsp finely grated ginger
2 tbsp sunflower seeds
green leaves of 2 spring onions
     (scallions), finely sliced
¼ red (bell) pepper or ¼ mild red
     chilli, finely sliced
1 tbsp soy sauce,
     plus more to serve
1 tbsp chopped coriander
     (cilantro) leaves

Place the rice noodles in a bowl and cover with boiling water. Let them soak for 5 minutes until they are soft, then drain.

Spiralise the courgettes, or cut them into strips with a julienne cutter.

Warm the oil in a spacious wok, drop in the sliced garlic and cook until it just begins to colour. Remove the garlic from the oil and discard it.

Add the ginger, sunflower seeds, spring onion greens and pepper, or chilli, and cook gently for a minute. Add the courgetti and stir-fry until the vegetables are soft but retain some 'bite'.

Add the drained noodles and continue to stir-fry. When the noodles have warmed through, add the soy sauce and serve strewn with a little chopped coriander and more soy sauce if required.

TRY THIS:
Serve with buckwheat noodles or black rice.

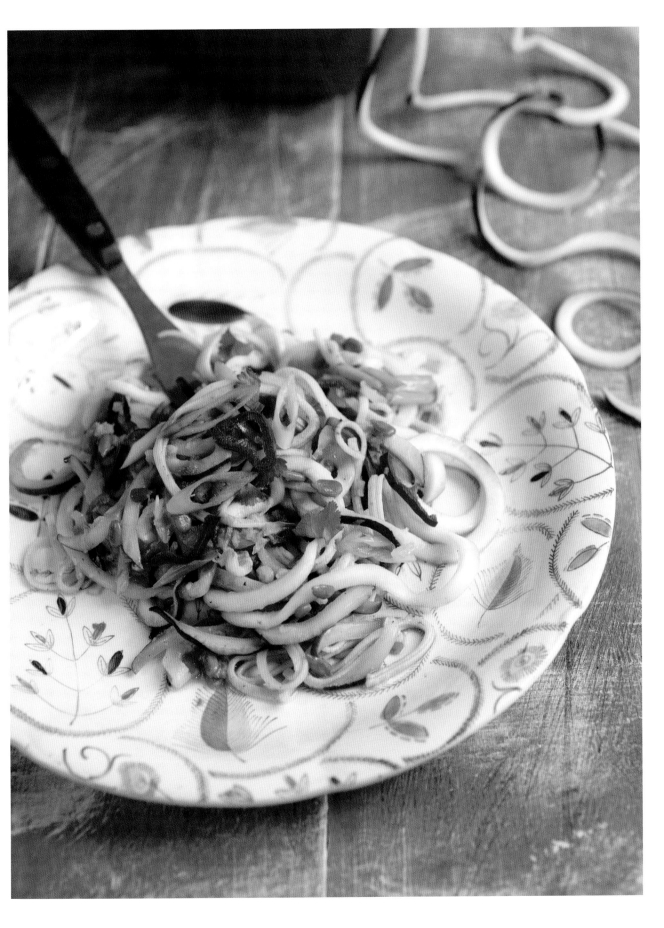

SIDE DISHES

Potato, rice and polenta are great ingredients to use for side dishes. Each recipe provides a useful source of energy and is suitable for a sensitive gut. These side dishes can be mixed and matched with the main dishes and help to complete the nutritional balance of a meal.

Basmati rice is a store cupboard staple and is quick to cook, whilst potatoes are endlessly versatile. Polenta is worth experimenting with and can taste very good with the addition of herbs and a little cheese. These side dishes should be as enjoyable as the main course itself.

Lemon rice with coriander and mustard seeds

Our favourite rice is basmati. It has a distinct fragrance and it cooks more quickly than other rice. This is a flavoursome side dish that goes so well with Herby fish cakes in tomato sauce (see p.83). It could even make a main course if you added a few stir-fried prawns and sliced vegetables.

SERVES 4
Hands-on time 5 minutes
Cooking time 12 minutes

175 g/6 oz/1 cup basmati rice
½ tsp sea salt and freshly ground
   black pepper
1 tbsp peanut
   or other flavourless oil
1 tbsp mustard seeds
3 tbsp chopped coriander
   (cilantro) leaves
finely grated zest and juice
   of ½ lemon

Pour the rice into a measuring jug and make a note of its volume. Place in a small saucepan with twice its volume of water and the ½ tsp of salt. Bring to the boil, cover with a tight-fitting lid and leave to simmer quietly on a very low heat for exactly 12 minutes. Continue to cook according to the directions for cooking rice (see p.41).

Gently heat the oil in a small frying pan, add the mustard seeds and cook until they pop.

Stir the coriander, mustard seeds and lemon zest and juice into the rice, season with salt and pepper, and serve.

Baked polenta with Gorgonzola and sage

This uses cooked polenta (see p.38), cut into fingers and baked until crisp. Adding sage and a strong-tasting blue cheese makes this humble dish special.

SERVES 4
Hands-on time 10 minutes
Cooking time 30 minutes

200 g/7 oz cooked and set
    polenta, cut into strips (see
    p.38)
2 tbsp olive oil
80 g/3 oz/¾ cup Gorgonzola
    cheese
5 sage leaves, finely chopped
sea salt and freshly ground
    black pepper

Preheat the oven to 200°C/400°F/gas 6.

Lay the polenta fingers on a lightly oiled baking tray and place in the oven to warm through and crisp for 25 minutes.

Crumble the Gorgonzola over the polenta. Scatter with the sage, salt and pepper, and return to the oven for 5 minutes for the cheese to melt.

Fennel and potato gratin

The long stems of the fennel herb are crowned with clusters of small flowers known as umbels, the leaves of which can be made into a soothing tea. The seeds have traditionally been used to soothe symptoms in the gut but do contain fructo-oligosaccharides (FOS), so don't eat too many. The green fronds can be used as a herb when cooking fish and making stock.

In this recipe, a bulb of fennel is finely sliced, layered with potato and baked with a crust of Parmesan cheese.

Often potato gratins contain garlic, but in this recipe fresh-picked chives work really well, and so does wild garlic, if it is in season.

SERVES 4
Hands-on time 10 minutes
Cooking time 40 minutes

1 small bulb of fennel, thinly
    sliced lengthways
sea salt and freshly ground
    black pepper
30 g/1 oz/2 tbsp unsalted butter
2 small floury potatoes, peeled,
    thinly shaved with a
    potato peeler
2 tsp chopped chives
100 ml/3 fl oz/½ cup lactose-free
    milk
60 g/2 oz/⅔ cup Parmesan
    cheese, finely grated

Preheat the oven to 200°C/400°F/gas 6. Place the sliced fennel in a pan of lightly salted water and boil for 5 minutes until tender. Drain the fennel, reserving 150 ml/5 fl oz/⅔ cup of the cooking water.

Lightly butter a baking dish and layer the sliced potatoes and fennel. Season the layers with a little salt and pepper and a scattering of chives. Mix the reserved cooking water and the milk together and pour over the potatoes and fennel, then dot a little butter over the surface and season with salt and pepper. Cover the gratin with foil.

Place the gratin on a baking tray to catch any spills and cook for 30 minutes. Remove the foil, scatter with the cheese, and cook for a further 10 minutes or until the vegetables are tender and the top begins to brown.

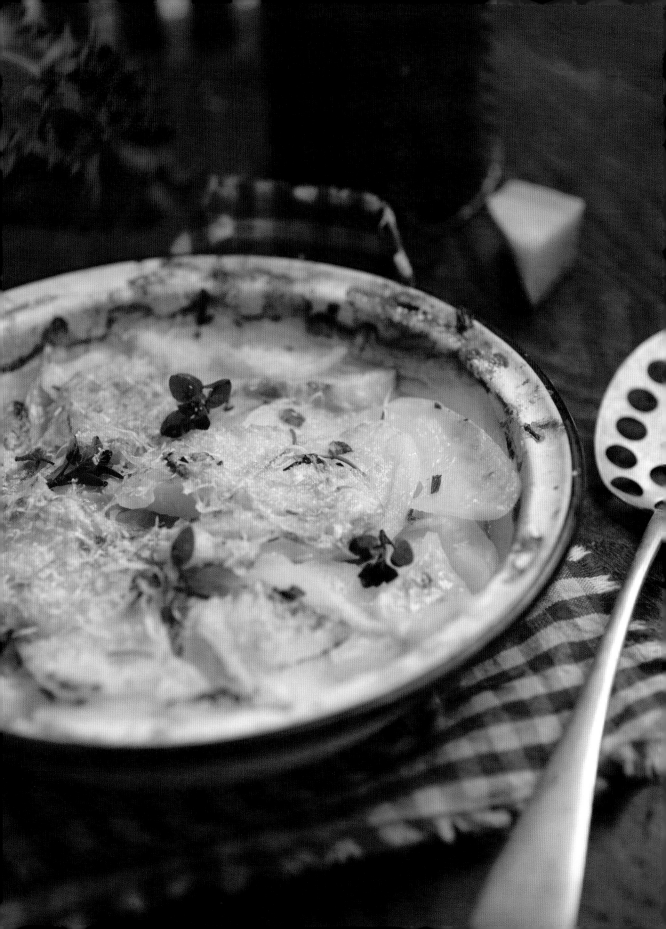

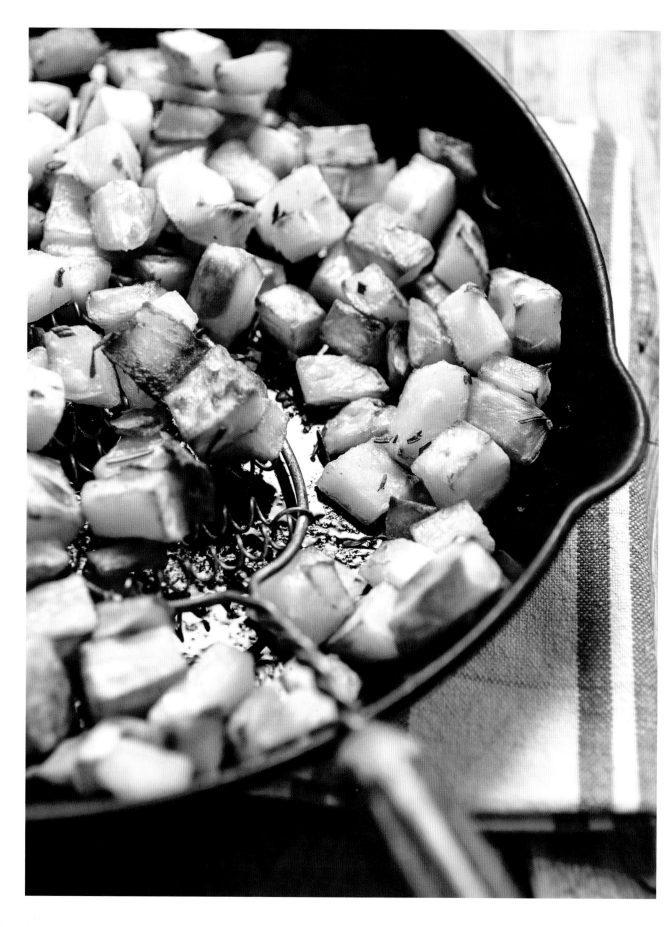

Oven-baked potatoes with rosemary and garlic oil

This is one of our favourite ways to eat potatoes. They can be cooking in the oven while you prepare the main dish, and you can make it with peeled potatoes or leave the skins on.

The combination of chopped rosemary, garlic oil and flaked sea salt elevate this to something special to go alongside a simple piece of grilled fish or meat. It would go well with Cod parcels with sauce vierge (see p.88) or Hot-smoked salmon with spinach and lemon (see p.73).

SERVES 4
Hands-on time 20 minutes
Cooking time 40 minutes

3 tbsp olive oil
2 garlic cloves, sliced
4 medium floury potatoes,
   scrubbed, cut into
   2 cm/1 in cubes
flaked sea salt
1 tbsp chopped rosemary

Preheat the oven to 200°C/400°F/gas 6.

Heat the olive oil in a small saucepan. Gently fry the garlic until beginning to brown. Discard the garlic and pour the oil into a large cast-iron pan, or roasting tin. Add the potatoes, sprinkle with salt and toss them in the garlic-flavoured oil.

Place the potatoes in the hot oven and, after 15 minutes, shuffle them around a bit to ensure they are cooking evenly. Return to the oven for a further 20 minutes, then scatter with the rosemary and a little more salt. Return the potatoes to the oven for another few minutes until golden brown and crisp.

PUDDINGS AND CAKES

Most of us like to eat something sweet to finish off a meal, or perhaps as a snack in the afternoon with a cup of tea. Although it is so much easier to buy a ready-made cake or dessert, the FODMAPs and fat content may not suit you. If you make your own, you'll know exactly what's in it.

Most of our puddings and cakes are simple and quick to make, but you need to be careful of ingredients and choose modest portion sizes, however tasty.

Adding fruit and vegetables to cakes can improve the texture by adding moisture and means less fat needs to be used. Many fruits can be tolerated by people with sensitive guts. For our recipes, we have selected only those in the green category from our guide in gut-friendly ingredients (see p.33). If your gut is particularly sensitive, no more than the equivalent of one piece of fruit should be included in a portion of pudding or cake, but you may be able to eat a little more when you feel better.

Puddings and cakes often contain wheat flour, which may trigger gut symptoms. But we have got round this by using gluten-free flours and ground nuts.

Passion fruit and raspberry mini pavlovas

Pavlova is a meringue-based dessert named after the Russian ballerina Anna Pavlova. The light-as-air white discs are reminiscent of the frothy petticoats of a ballerina's skirts, and this is a foolproof method to make them: whisking the egg whites over hot water causes the air inside the bubbles to expand and makes the meringue light and easy to shape.

A little whipped cream can be eaten by most people who are intolerant to lactose.

SERVES 4
Hands-on time 15 minutes
Cooking time 45 minutes

150 g/5 oz (about 4 large) egg
   whites
about 300 g/10 oz/1½ cups
   caster (superfine) sugar
200 ml/7 fl oz/¾ cup double
   (heavy) cream
100 g/3½ oz/1 cup raspberries
4 passion fruits, halved, insides
   scooped out
edible flowers, such as daisies,
   violas, marigolds or nasturtiums
   (optional)

Preheat the oven to 110°C/225°F/gas ¼.

Check the weight of the egg whites and then weigh exactly double their weight of caster sugar. Place the egg whites and sugar in a heatproof bowl over a pan of simmering water. Make sure the base of the bowl does not touch the water. Using an electric mixer, whisk the egg whites until the sugar has dissolved; you can test this by dipping 2 clean fingers into the mixture and rubbing them together. If you can still feel sugar crystals, mix for a little longer. Whisk the meringue a little more until it is stiff and glossy. This usually takes about 5 minutes. Remove the bowl from the heat, taking care to protect your hands with some oven gloves.

Line 2 baking trays with baking parchment. Arrange spoons of meringue on the baking parchment, leaving plenty of space between each. Flatten each blob of meringue into a circle about 10 cm/4 in across. Put both trays into the preheated oven and bake for about 45 minutes or until the outside is set like a shell; it will remain a little soft inside. Allow to cool.

Whip the cream to soft peaks. Spread a little whipped cream over the base of a meringue and top with the raspberries and the pulp and seeds from the passion fruits. Carefully place the other meringue on top. Decorate with clean, untreated edible flowers, if you have them.

Coconut frozen yogurt with pine nuts and cocoa nibs

This uses a dairy-free yogurt made from coconut milk that has been inoculated with live probiotic cultures. If you cannot find yogurt made from coconut milk, you can use yogurt flavoured with coconut. The tropical coconut flavour matches banana perfectly and this frozen yogurt is lower in fat than regular ice cream. It can be dressed up with chocolate, cocoa nibs and pine nuts to make a stylish pudding, or served as it is.

SERVES 4
Hands-on time 10 minutes,
    plus 2 hours for freezing

FOR THE FROZEN YOGURT
200 g/7 oz/¾ cup coconut yogurt
200 ml/7 fl oz/¾ cup coconut
    milk
½ tsp vanilla extract
1 large banana
1 tbsp maple syrup
    or golden syrup

TO SERVE
2 tbsp pine nuts
60 g/2 oz/½ cup dark chocolate
    (at least 60% cocoa solids),
    broken into pieces
1 tbsp cocoa nibs

Place the coconut yogurt, coconut milk, vanilla, banana and syrup in a liquidiser and process for a minute.

Churn the mixture in an ice cream maker and store following the manufacturor's instructions. If churning by hand, pour into a container with a lid and place in the freezer. After 1 hour, take the mixture from the freezer and mix vigorously with a fork to break up the ice crystals. Return to the freezer and freeze for another hour. If you have time, stir the frozen yogurt with a fork every 15 minutes; this will break up the ice crystals and give a smoother texture.

Heat a heavy-based frying pan and scatter the pine nuts evenly over the base. Cook them gently until just turning brown, shaking the pan to ensure they brown evenly.

Melt the chocolate in a heatproof bowl over a saucepan of hot water (the base of the bowl should not touch the water).

To serve, scoop the frozen yogurt into bowls, scatter with pine nuts and cocoa nibs and drizzle with melted chocolate.

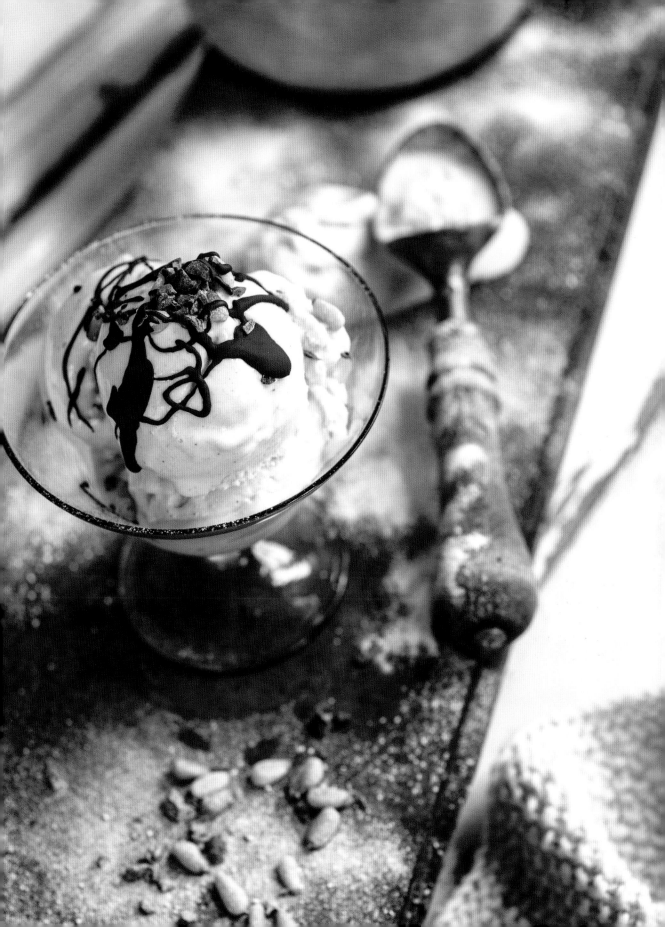

Chocolate pots with salted almond butter

This is a delightful recipe that can be eaten as an everyday treat or dressed up with fruit and an extra drizzle of melted chocolate for a special occasion. It is basically real custard made from egg yolks but, instead of using cow's milk, we have substituted almond milk. If your almond milk is already sweetened, you will need a little less maple syrup. You can use either almond butter or a good-quality natural peanut butter, both work well. The chocolate pots can be made a few hours before serving and are ideal to serve for a meal with friends.

We really like serving them in vintage tea cups; the cooking temperature is moderate and tea cups should withstand the heat. China ramekins can be used instead.

SERVES 4
Hands-on time 10 minutes
Cooking time 35 minutes

250 ml/9 fl oz/1 cup almond milk
½ tsp vanilla extract
2 tbsp almond butter (or good-
    quality peanut butter)
2 large egg yolks,
    at room temperature
2 tbsp maple syrup
    or golden syrup
pinch of sea salt
100 g/3½ oz/¾ cup dark
    chocolate (60% minimum cocoa
    solids), coarsely chopped
50 g/2 oz/½ cup raspberries,
    strawberries or blueberries
    to decorate

Preheat the oven to 150°C/300°F/gas 2.

In a small saucepan gently heat the almond milk, vanilla and almond butter. Stir a few times to make sure the almond butter melts into the milk.

Meanwhile, whisk together the egg yolks, maple syrup and sea salt in a mixing bowl.

Remove the milk from the heat, add the dark chocolate pieces and stir well to ensure the chocolate melts.

Pour the molten chocolate mixture over the egg yolks and continue to whisk. It is important to do this slowly, so the eggs do not coagulate.

Place 6 small china cups (or ramekins) inside a deep roasting tin filled halfway up with hot water. Pour the custard into the cups and carefully place the roasting tin on a rack inside the oven.

Bake for 30 minutes, or until set. You can test this by pressing gently on the surface of the chocolate pot.

Remove from the oven and cool completely before decorating with a few berries. The chocolate pots can be stored in the fridge for a few hours before serving.

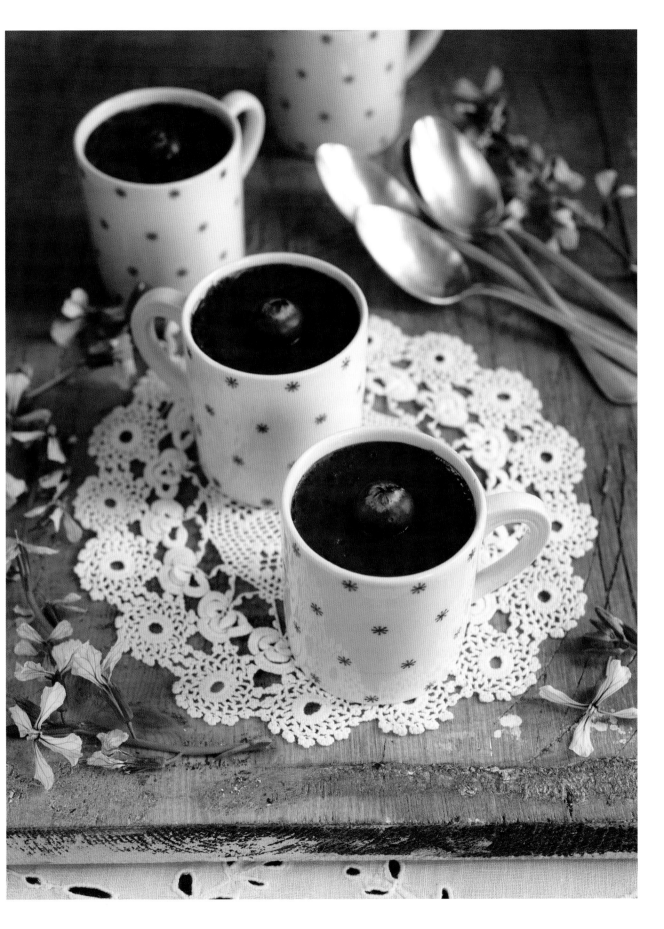

Blood orange granita

This is a spectacular pudding ideally suited to a warm day and so simple to make. Granita is made up of crunchy, large ice crystals and does not require much attention once you have juiced the oranges.

It is a great fat-free, big-flavoured convenient pudding that can sit happily in the freezer until needed. We have tried not to use too much sugar but, if you have a sweet tooth, you can adjust the sweetness to your taste.

Blood oranges are seasonal and this is a way of preserving their precious red juice to eat during the summer. They have a distinct 'sherbet' taste which is both sweet yet deliciously sour. Regular oranges can be used instead to make a delicious granita, but it doesn't look quite as amazing.

SERVES 4
Hands-on time 10 minutes
Cooking time 5 minutes,
    plus 4 hours freezing

150 g/5 oz/¾ cup caster
    (superfine) sugar
500 ml/18 fl oz/2 cups blood
    orange juice (about 6 oranges)
4 tbsp Campari or Cointreau
    (optional)

Place 150 ml/5 fl oz/⅔ cup of water in a saucepan and add the sugar. Bring to the boil and stir until the sugar has dissolved. Remove the syrup from the heat and cool. Chill thoroughly.

Place the orange juice in a bowl, add the chilled sugar syrup and stir. Pour into a plastic storage container, cover with a lid and freeze for at least 4 hours.

When ice crystals begin to form around the edge of the container, stir the granita with a fork every hour or so, paying special attention to the sides. You should end up with a gloriously slushy bright-red granita after about 6 hours.

Remove the granita from the freezer 10–15 minutes before serving. Scrape the frozen granita with a fork so that it takes on a slushy look and serve in glasses or small bowls.

Drizzle a little Campari or Cointreau over the granita just before serving, if you like.

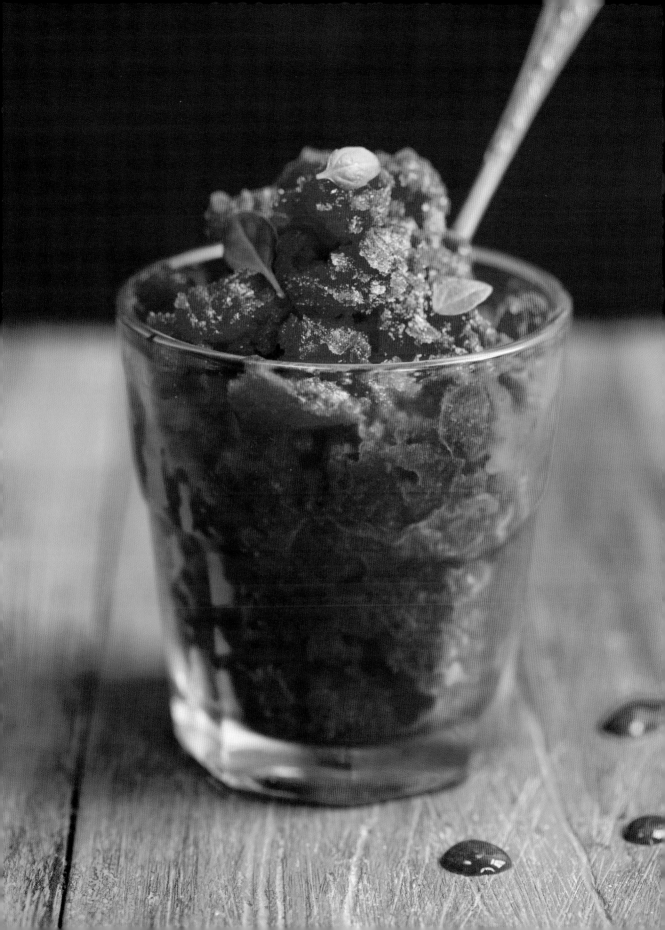

Blueberry Florentines

These sweet, buttery, gluten-free biscuits are one of the most luxurious things you can make. They are traditionally made with glacé cherries but we have substituted blueberries dried in the oven. Florentines look pretty and delicate, but the mixture is a devil in the oven as it tends to spread all over the baking sheet. Do not let that put you off! As it cools and hardens, bring it back into line with a biscuit cutter. You can even use your fingers to help shape any edges that don't look quite round.

MAKES ABOUT 24
Hands-on time 20 minutes
Cooking time 40 minutes

150 g/5 oz/¾ cup blueberries
1 tsp caster (superfine) sugar
100 g/3½ oz/1 stick unsalted butter
150 g/5 oz/¾ cup soft brown sugar
175 g/6 oz/⅔ cup golden syrup
100 g/3½ oz/¾ cup gluten-free flour
2 tsp ground ginger
150 g/5 oz/1½ cups mixed nuts, roughly crushed
150 g/5 oz/1¼ cups dark chocolate (60% minimum cocoa solids), broken into small pieces

Preheat the oven to 200°C/400°F/gas 6. Place the blueberries on a baking tray lined with non-stick baking parchment and sprinkle with the caster sugar. Bake for 20 minutes until almost dried out. Remove from the oven and set aside to cool.

To make the biscuits, place the butter, brown sugar and golden syrup in a saucepan and melt over a low heat. Stir in the flour and ginger.

Line 2 large baking trays with non-stick baking parchment and pour half the mixture on to the middle of one of the trays. Spread it out evenly over the tray using a palette knife or spatula. Leave a 2 cm/1 in gap around the mixture as it will spread while cooking. Repeat with the remaining mixture.

Place both trays in the oven and cook for 5 minutes. The mixture may look unpromising at this stage as it will have spread a lot, but do not worry. Sprinkle the crushed nuts over and scatter with the dried blueberries. Return to the oven and cook for 10–15 minutes until bubbling and golden brown. Remove from the oven and set aside to cool for 5–10 minutes.

Cut out discs with a biscuit cutter as the mixture begins to set. Remove to a plate and allow the Florentines to cool and harden in the fridge. The offcuts should be allowed to set, then broken up and kept in an airtight container. They are delicious over yogurt or added to a crumble mix.

Half-fill a small saucepan with water and bring to a simmer. Place the chocolate pieces in a small heatproof bowl over the saucepan of hot water (the base of the bowl should not touch the water) and stir the chocolate until it melts.

Remove the Florentines from the fridge and either dip each into the melted chocolate or drizzle with melted chocolate. Place on non-stick baking parchment on a tray and cool in the fridge to set.

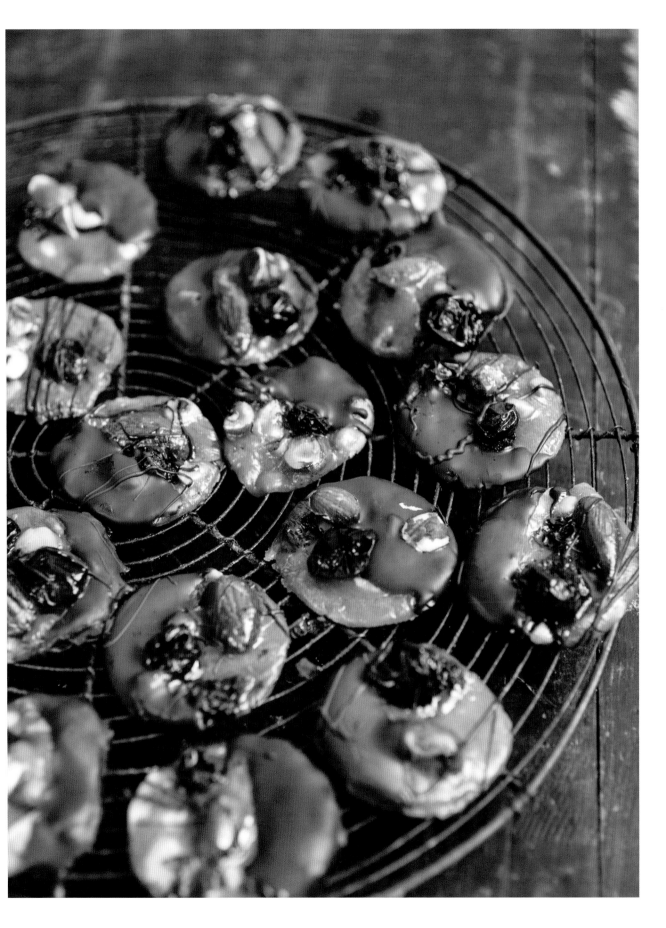

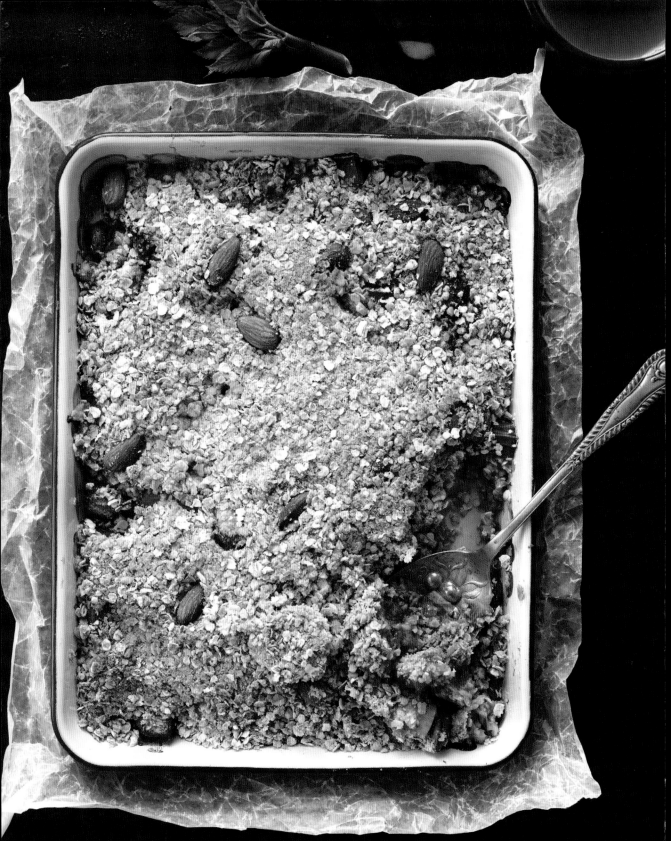

Rhubarb and strawberry crumble

Crumbles are a great way to use up seasonal fruit. Sadly apples, pears and stone fruits do not suit people with a sensitive gut, but there is another option. Rhubarb is perfect as it yields beautiful juices when cooked and can be teamed up with other delicious, soothing ingredients such as strawberries or ginger, both of which are fine. The best rhubarb to use in puddings is young, forced, pink-stemmed rhubarb, which is in the shops in the UK from January for a couple of months. This is the most flavoursome and tender rhubarb to use. If you make this dish in spring, be sure to add some sweet cicely, if you can, because its flavour-enhancing qualities means you can use less sugar.

SERVES 4
Hands-on time 15 minutes
Cooking time 20 minutes

FOR THE FILLING
400 g/14 oz/4 cups rhubarb, cut
    into 2 cm/1 in lengths
400 g/14 oz/3 cups strawberries,
    quartered
finely grated zest and juice of
    1 lemon
3 tbsp caster (superfine) sugar

FOR THE CRUMBLE
75 g/3 oz/¾ cup rolled oats
60 g/2 oz/½ cup buckwheat flour
pinch of sea salt
40 g/1½ oz/¼ cup soft brown
    sugar
½ tsp vanilla extract
40 g/1½ oz/3 tbsp coconut oil
1 tbsp chopped nuts, such as
    almonds, pecans or walnuts
1 tbsp pumpkin seeds

Preheat the oven to 190°C/375°F/gas 5. Place the rhubarb, strawberries, lemon zest and juice and sugar in a bowl and mix well. Set aside.

Prepare the crumble. Mix the oats, buckwheat flour and salt in a bowl. Stir in the sugar, vanilla and coconut oil, and mix with your hands. Scatter the nuts and seeds into the crumble mix.

Place the fruit in a baking tin measuring about 25 x 20 cm (10 x 8 in) and spread the crumble on top. Bake for 30 minutes until the top is golden brown and the juice from the fruit is bubbling through the crumble.

Lemon and cardamom polenta cake

We love this gluten-free cake. It is moist, syrupy and fragrant, quick to make and created from low-FODMAPs ingredients. If you need to make your own ground almonds from whole almonds, soak them in boiling water for a minute. Remove the almonds from the water with a slotted spoon and slip off their skins. Allow any remaining water to evaporate from the surface of the almonds before grinding them in a coffee mill or food processor.

SERVES 12
Hands-on time 10 minutes
Cooking time 40 minutes

FOR THE CAKE
45 g/1½ oz/¼ cup polenta
200 g/7 oz/1 cup golden caster (superfine) sugar
100 g/3½ oz/1 cup ground almonds (almond flour)
finely grated zest of 1 orange
finely grated zest of 1 lemon
1½ tsp baking powder
4 eggs, lightly beaten
200 ml/7 fl oz/1 cup light vegetable oil, such as sunflower or rapeseed

FOR THE SYRUP
55 g/2 oz/¼ cup granulated sugar
juice of 1 orange
juice of 1 lemon
2 cinnamon sticks
3 star anise
5 cardamom pods
2 tbsp icing sugar

Line a cake tin measuring 23 cm/9 in across and 7 cm/3 in deep with non-stick baking parchment. Combine the polenta, caster sugar, ground almonds, zests and baking powder in a large bowl. Whisk the eggs and oil together and gradually beat these into the dry ingredients with a wooden spoon to form a thick batter.

Position the cake tin on a baking tray and fill it with the batter.

Place in a cold oven and set it at 190°C/375°F/gas 5. Bake the cake for 40 minutes or until it is golden brown and a skewer can be inserted and removed clean from its centre.

Remove the cake from the oven and cool for 5 minutes.

Meanwhile, for the syrup, boil the granulated sugar and juices with the cinnamon sticks, star anise and cardamom pods. Simmer for 5 minutes, stirring to dissolve the sugar. Remove the spices and set aside.

With a skewer, stab the cake all over to create soaking holes for the syrup. Pour the spiced syrup over the cake while it is cooling. Use the strained-out spices to decorate the cake.

When the cake is cold, turn out of the tin and place, spice-side up, on a serving plate (be careful as this is tricky and sticky!). Sift over the icing sugar and serve.

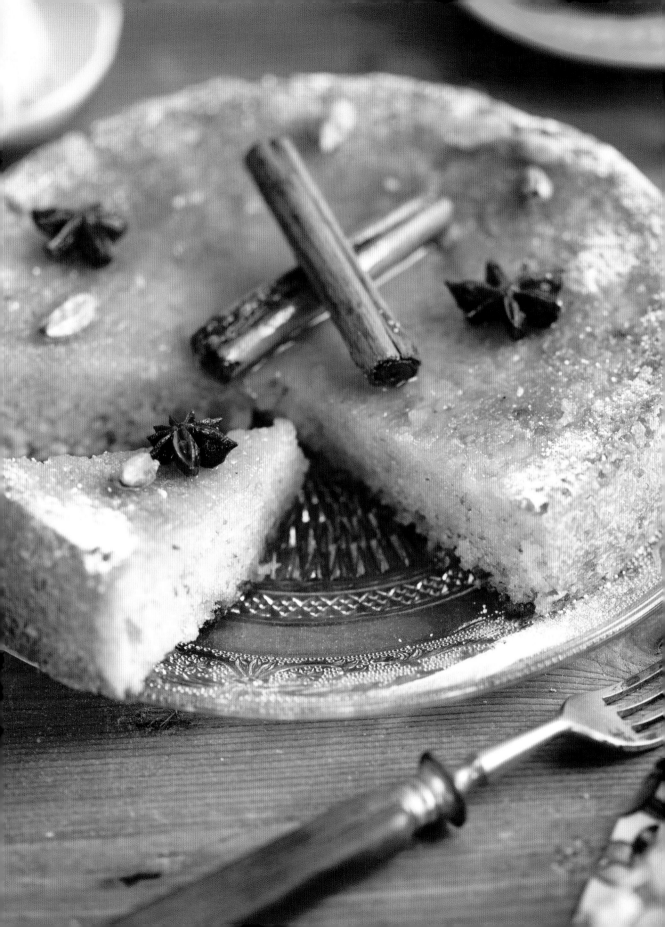

Chocolate, aubergine and cranberry cake

This cake has a festive air and could be served at Christmas or another wintry celebration. Few people will guess it contains aubergine. The cooked aubergine replaces the fat usually found in cakes and adds moisture and a silky smooth texture. But don't be fooled into thinking this cake is low fat. Just 100 g/3½ oz chocolate contains about 30 g/1 oz of fat, so just eat a small piece of this and share the rest of the cake around.

MAKES 15 SLICES
OR 15 CUP CAKES
Hands-on time 20 minutes
Cooking time 40 minutes

a little oil, for the tin
    (if making 1 large cake)
1 large aubergine (weighing
    roughly 400 g/14 oz)
300 g/10 oz/2½ cups dark
    chocolate (60% minimum
    cocoa solids), broken
    into squares
50 g/2 oz/⅓ cup cocoa powder
50 g/2 oz/¼ cup ground almonds
    (almond flour)
3 medium eggs
1 tsp orange extract
finely grated zest of 1 orange
200 g/7 oz/⅔ cup golden syrup
2 tsp baking powder
pinch of sea salt
1 tbsp brandy
100 g/4 oz/½ cup fresh or frozen
    cranberries
1 tbsp caster (superfine) sugar

Preheat the oven to 180°C/350°C/gas 4. To make one cake, you will need a loose-based cake tin 23 cm/9 in in diameter and 7 cm/3 in deep, or for small cakes a 12-hole cake or muffin tray.

Line the cake tin with non-stick baking parchment and brush lightly with oil. Or fill the muffin tin with small paper muffin cases.

Puncture the aubergine all over with a skewer, place in a bowl, cover with cling film (plastic wrap) and cook in a microwave on high for 5 minutes until soft. Throw away any liquid that has accumulated and leave to cool a little.

Skin the aubergine and purée with a stick blender or liquidiser. Add the broken-up chocolate, which will melt in the warmth of the aubergine. Place the remaining ingredients apart from the cranberries and caster sugar in a large bowl and mix thoroughly. Stir in the aubergine mixture and half the cranberries.

Pour into the prepared tin or cases and bake a large cake for 40 minutes and small cakes for 20 minutes.

Remove from the oven and cool for 15 minutes before turning out on to a cooling tray.

Place the remaining cranberries in a small bowl with the caster sugar and cook in the microwave on high for 1 minute. Use these to decorate the cake(s).

TRY THIS:
Substitute raspberries for cranberries: perfect for summer.

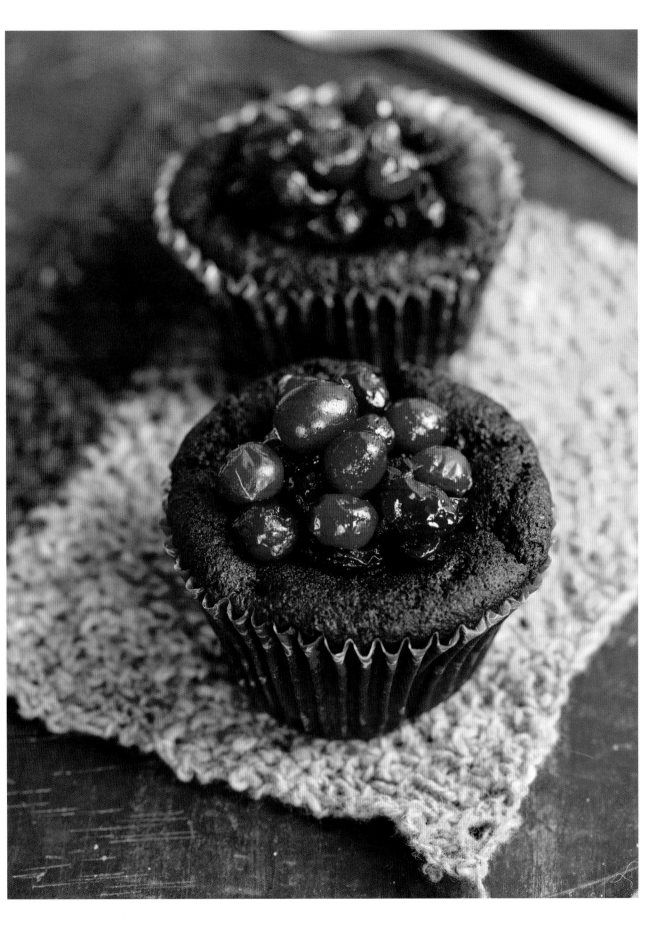

Banana, vanilla and pecan nut cake

We had been looking for a reliable, light, flavoursome cake for ages but couldn't find one. So we formulated this stunning recipe out of the contents of the store cupboard. It is made with gluten-free flour and ground almonds, but the really special thing is the flavour of banana coupled with vanilla and pecan nuts. It tastes gorgeous fresh out of the oven and the texture is perfect: light and fluffy.

SERVES 8
Hands-on time 15 minutes
Cooking time 50 minutes

FOR THE CAKE
125 g/4½ oz soft unsalted butter,
    plus more for the tin
125 g/4½ oz/²/₃ cup soft brown
    sugar
2 eggs, lightly beaten, at room
    temperature
75 g/3 oz/½ cup plain white
    gluten-free flour
¾ tsp baking powder
75 g/3 oz/¾ cup ground almonds
    (almond flour)
2 small ripe bananas, mashed
1 tsp vanilla extract
60 g/2 oz/½ cup pecan nut pieces

FOR THE ICING
100 g/3½ oz/¾ cup white
    chocolate, broken into pieces
350 g/12 oz/2²/₃ cups icing
    (confectioner's) sugar
1½ tbsp unsalted butter
½ tsp vanilla extract
a little lactose-free milk, if needed

TO DECORATE
30 g/1 oz/⅓ cup pecan nuts,
    dry roasted in a pan

Preheat the oven to 190°C/375°F/gas 5. Butter and line a small loaf tin measuring 20 x 10 cm/8 x 4 in with silicone baking paper or a cake liner.

Beat the butter and brown sugar together until paler and fluffy. Gradually beat in the eggs a little at a time.

Sift together the flour and baking powder, and fold these into the butter mixture. Fold in the ground almonds, bananas, vanilla and pecan nuts. Spoon into the prepared tin.

Bake the cake for 50 minutes. To see if it is done, insert a skewer into the centre; it should come out clean. Remove from the tin and place on a cooling rack.

For the icing, melt the white chocolate in a heatproof bowl over a pan of simmering water (don't let the base of the bowl touch the water). Leave to cool slightly. Beat the icing sugar, butter, vanilla and white chocolate together until you have a thick icing. (Add a little milk if you need to loosen the icing.) Spread over the banana cake and decorate with toasted pecan nuts.

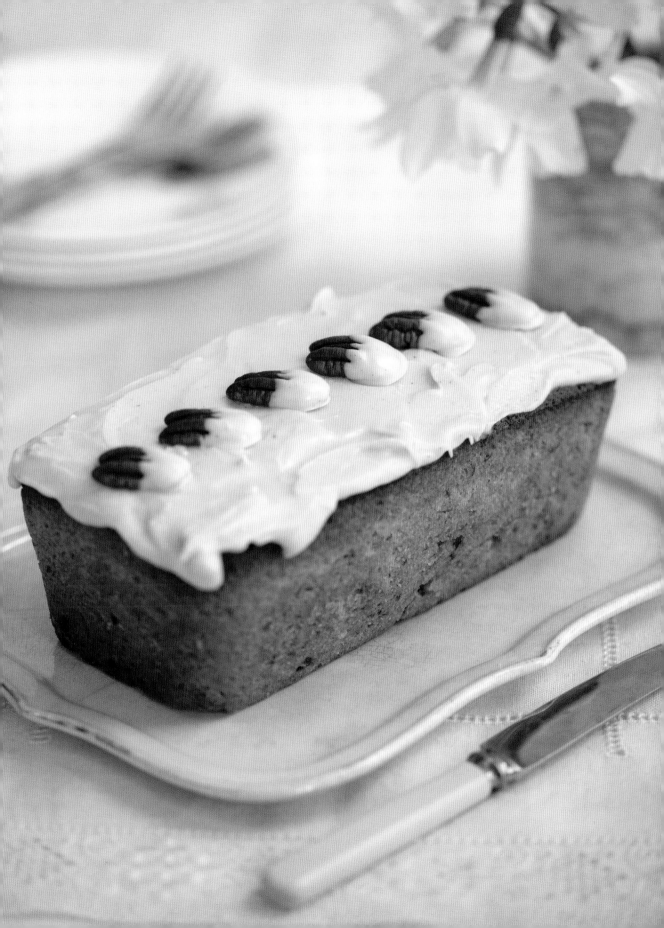

Flapjack with coconut oil, nuts and seeds

Flapjacks are an old favourite, but most recipes contain a lot of fat. This is one of the best we have tasted and this version has been brought up to date. By using melted coconut oil, we use less fat than comparable recipes, as only a small amount is needed to bind the nuts, seeds and oats together. It also gives a great flavour.

The beauty of these little bars is their portability. Just wrap in waxed paper or foil and take them with you if you are pushed for time and can't eat breakfast at home.

MAKES 12
Hands-on time 10 minutes
Cooking time 25 minutes

200 g/7 oz/2 cups rolled oats
60 g/2 oz/½ cup nuts, walnuts,
    hazelnuts or macadamia,
    roughly chopped
2 tbsp sunflower seeds
2 tbsp poppy seeds
2 tbsp pumpkin seeds
1 tbsp chia seeds, mixed with
    2 tbsp cold water
2 tbsp raisins
60 g/2 oz/⅓ cup soft brown sugar
2 tbsp golden syrup
60 g/2 oz/⅓ cup coconut oil

Preheat the oven to 180°C/350°F/gas 4. Line a 30 x 20 cm (12 x 8 in) and 2.5 cm/1 in deep baking tray with baking parchment, cutting slits in each corner so it fits more neatly.

Mix the oats, nuts and dry seeds together in a bowl and stir in the chia seeds and raisins.

Place the soft brown sugar, golden syrup and coconut oil in a small saucepan and heat gently until the sugar has dissolved and the coconut oil has melted. Remove from the heat and stir into the oat mixture. Mix well.

Transfer the mixture to the prepared tray and press down firmly with a palette knife or the back of a metal spoon. The oat mixture should be about 2 cm/¾ in thick and cover half the baking tray.

Bake for 25 minutes until it begins to turn golden brown at the edges. Do not let it overcook. The flapjack will still be soft at this point. Remove the baking tray from the oven.

Allow the flapjack to cool a little before cutting into 12 small rectangles while it is still warm. As it continues to cool, it will harden. Store the bars in an airtight container for up to a week.

Spiced carrot, orange and quinoa cake

This is a gluten-free cake made with ingredients that should not trigger symptoms. It is quick to make, low in fat and has a moist, flavoursome bite. Quinoa is usually associated with savoury dishes, but it can be put to good use in sweet recipes, too. In this recipe, we use it to replace flour. The quinoa needs to be cooked in advance, according to the packet instructions (usually 8 minutes in boiling water).

SERVES 12
Hands-on time 15 minutes
Cooking time 45 minutes

FOR THE CAKE
170 g/5½ oz/scant 1 cup quinoa
100 g/3½ oz/¾ cup gluten-free
    self-raising (self-rising) flour
175 g/6 oz/1¾ cups ground
    almonds (almond flour)
100 g/3½ oz/1 cup walnuts,
    roughly chopped
1½ tsp ground coriander seeds
1½ tsp ground cinnamon
½ tsp mixed spice
100 g/3½ oz/⅔ cup light brown
    sugar
185 ml/6 fl oz/¾ cup sunflower oil
3 eggs, lightly beaten
80 g/3 oz/¼ cup golden or
    maple syrup
250 g/9 oz/3 cups carrots, grated

FOR THE TOPPING (OPTIONAL)
80 g/3 oz/⅔ cup dark chocolate
    (60% minimum cocoa solids),
    broken into pieces
25 g/1 oz/1½ tbsp good-quality
    or home-made candied peel

Preheat the oven to 180°C/350°F/gas 4. Line a 23 cm/9 in diameter cake tin with non-stick baking paper.

Boil the quinoa for 10 minutes, or according to the packet instructions, then drain.

Place the flour, ground almonds, walnuts, spices and light brown sugar in a bowl and mix thoroughly. This is the dry mixture.

Combine the oil, eggs and syrup in a large bowl and process together with a stick blender or a hand whisk. This is the wet mixture.

Add the wet mixture to the dry mixture and stir in the quinoa and carrots. Fold together carefully until well combined.

Spoon into the prepared tin and bake for 45 minutes or until just turning golden brown; it should be springy to the touch. Remove the cake from the oven and, when cool enough, release it from the tin and allow it to cool completely.

To decorate the cake, put the chocolate in a heatproof bowl over hot water and allow it to melt (the base of the bowl should not touch the water). Drizzle the top of the cake with the melted chocolate and decorate with candied orange peel. Or you could simply dust the cake with a little sifted icing sugar.

DRINKS

The amount of fluid you need depends on many things, including the weather, how much physical activity you do and your age, but women need about 1.6 litres (nearly 3 pints/ 1.5 quarts) and men need about 2 litres (3 ½ pints/2 quarts) every day. This is on top of the water provided by the food you eat. You can top up your fluid levels from nearly all fluid that you drink, apart from alcoholic drinks.

You *could* just drink water, but how much more interesting and refreshing it is to make up your own drinks from fruit and vegetables. With their vibrant, enticing colours and clean, fresh flavours, a juice or smoothie can provide nutrients without feeling overwhelming, as the constituent parts might seem if they were solid. As always, the trick is to use a mix of fruit and vegetables that will be soothing to the gut.

There are just a few things to note. If you juice fruit and vegetables, most of the fibre is removed and you are left with a more concentrated version than if you ate the fruit or vegetable whole; that might trigger symptoms in some people. So our advice is to drink only a small glass (250 ml/9 fl oz/ 1 cup) and dilute it with a little water. Making smoothies, on the other hand, retains fibre, so most people with a sensitive gut should be able to tolerate the recommended portion of fruit in the form of a smoothie.

A glass of good wine with a meal is a lovely way to relax, but too much can cause dehydration and may well irritate and upset your gut.

Pineapple and coconut shake

The combination of pineapple and coconut makes good use of two ingredients to make a nutritious shake that can fill a gap if you don't feel like a full meal.

We have used bee pollen to add a few more nutrients and interest to this smoothie. Pollen is the bees' source of protein and is collected by beekeepers in a small pollen trap on the entrance of the hive. It is not an essential ingredient, but it is rather beautiful and tastes really lovely.

SERVES 4
Hands-on time 5 minutes

300 g/10 oz/1⅓ cups pineapple, chopped
3 tbsp coconut yogurt, or plain yogurt
400 ml/14 fl oz/1⅔ cups almond milk
1 banana
1 tbsp oats
1 tsp bee pollen (optional)
a few mint leaves, shredded

Place the first 5 ingredients into a tall jug and liquidise with a stick blender. Pour into 4 glasses and scatter with bee pollen and shredded mint leaves.

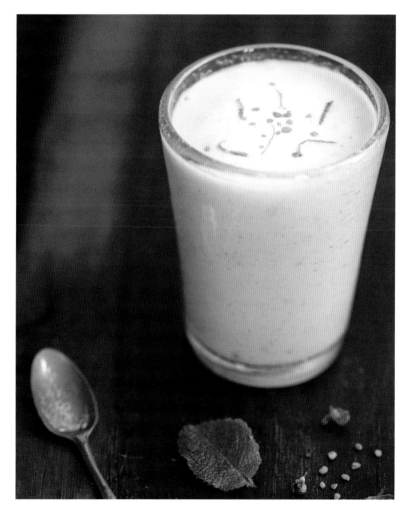

Green winter juice

This is a great drink that can be tweaked according to the ingredients you have in your fridge. If you do not have parsley, you can add a little more spinach. A kiwi fruit could be added to the mix, if you have one to use up.

SERVES 4
Hands-on time 5 minutes

1 lime, halved
1 orange, halved
1 lemongrass stalk
¾ cucumber
4 handfuls of spinach leaves
1–2 sprigs parsley
150 ml/ 5 fl oz/⅔ cup cold water
small bowl of crushed ice

Juice the lime and orange in a citrus press and reserve in a jug.

Roughly chop the lemongrass and cucumber, and feed them through the chute of a juicer. You do not get much juice from lemongrass but the flavour is intense and goes a long way to flavouring the juice. Add to the jug.

Feed the spinach and parsley through the juicer followed by the cold water. Add the green juice to the jug, stir together and serve.

Blueberry smoothie

This is a delicious, nutritious smoothie that is quick to make if you are pinched for time and need a snack or pick-me-up.

SERVES 4
Hands-on time 5 minutes

150 g/5 oz/¾ cup blueberries,
   fresh or frozen
juice of ½ lime
500 ml/18 fl oz/2 cups plant milk,
   such as almond, oat or rice
2 bananas
1 tbsp good-quality nut butter,
   such as almond or peanut
crushed ice, to serve

Pulse the blueberries and lime juice with a stick blender and divide between 4 glasses. Liquidise the plant milk, bananas and peanut butter with the stick blender and pour over the blueberry and lime juice. Stir in some crushed ice and serve with a straw.

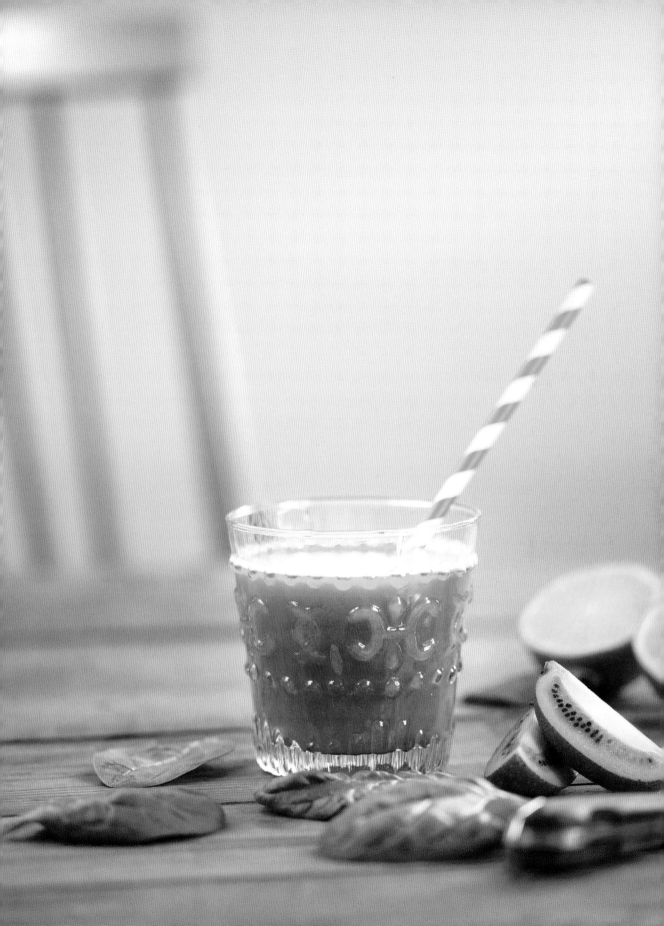

Carrot and ginger juice

The flavours of carrot and ginger suit each other well. Ginger is slightly hot and spicy and lifts the earthy flavour of carrot. Ginger is also very soothing for a sensitive gut. Juicing fruit concentrates the nutrients and the natural sugars present in the carrots, so it is important to dilute the juice with a little water. The bright orange colour is due to the rich quantities of beta carotenes present in carrots. Beta carotene gets converted to vitamin A in the body.

SERVES 4
Hands-on time 5 minutes

1 tbsp lemon juice
300 g/10 oz/1¼ cups carrots, peeled and roughly chopped
60 g/2 oz root ginger, or to taste
200 ml/7 fl oz/¾ cup ice-cold water

Put lemon juice in a jug; this will stop the carrot juice from discolouring. Feed the carrots through the juicer and collect the juice in the jug containing the lemon juice. Feed half the ginger through the juicer, mix it with the carrot juice and taste the juice to check the flavour is to your liking. Add more ginger as you prefer. This quantity of carrots and ginger should yield about 200 ml/7 fl oz/¾ cup juice. Dilute this juice with equal quantities of cold water and serve.

Raspberry shake

Combining plant milk with fruit makes a filling and hydrating drink, rich in nutrients. Other fruits such as banana, blueberries and strawberries can be used as a substitute for raspberries.

MAKES 4 SMALL SERVINGS
Hands-on time 5 minutes

300 g/10 oz/2 generous cups raspberries
570 ml/1 pint/2¼ cups lactose-free cow's milk, or almond, oat or rice milk
2 tbsp Greek yogurt

Place the raspberries, milk and yogurt in a liquidiser and process for 30 seconds until all the raspberries have been broken down to form a smooth drink.

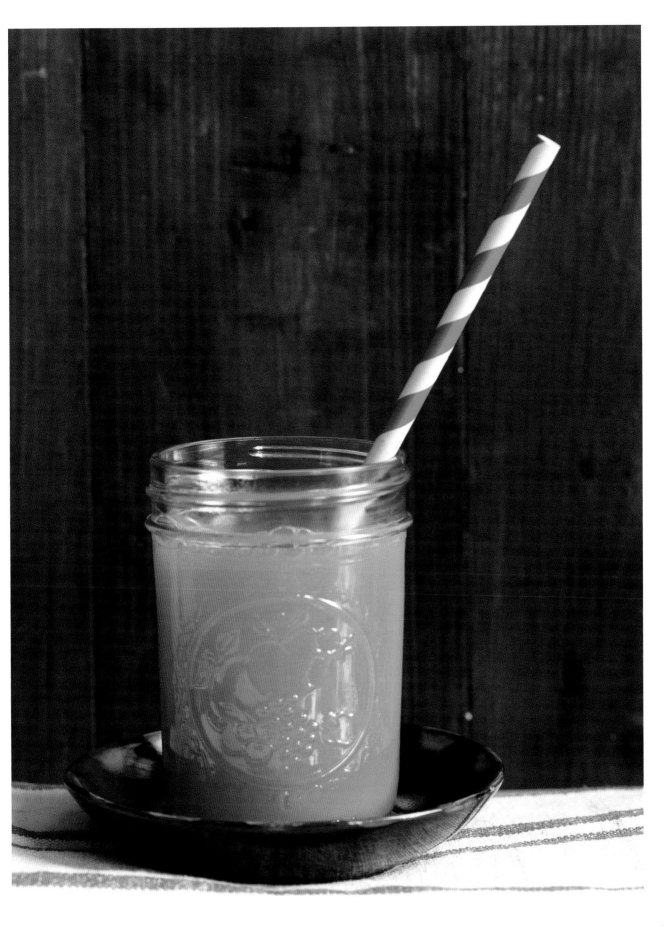

Elderflower lemonade

The sweetly scented lacy-cream flowers of elder appear in the hedgerows, wasteland and scrubby woods in abundance in the early weeks of summer. The fresh flowers make beguiling aromatic lemonade. They are best gathered just as they begin to open, as older flowers lose their perfume. The scent of the flowers differs between trees, and it is important to take the time to sniff out the one you like best. Spare a few elderflowers as they are needed to produce berries later, so pick from lots of different trees if possible. Elderflowers can be frozen for use later in drinks and puddings. Gathering elderflowers is a wonderfully relaxing activity that you can combine with a gentle walk on a fine day in early summer.

MAKES 2 LITRES/3½ PINTS/
2 GENEROUS QUARTS
Hands-on time 30 minutes, plus
   elderflower picking!

30 large elderflower heads,
   collected on a dry day
3 lemons, cut into thin slices
250 g/9 oz caster (superfine)
   sugar

Shake the elderflower heads to make sure they are free of any bugs. Arrange the flower heads and lemon slices in a large, heatproof bowl or bucket. Bring 2 litres/3½ pints/2 generous quarts of water to boil in a saucepan. Add the sugar to the water and stir until it has dissolved. Pour the sugar and water solution over the elderflowers and sliced lemons.

Cover loosely and leave to steep somewhere cool for 2 days. The longer you leave them, the stronger the flavour will become.

Place a double layer of muslin or cheesecloth over a bowl and strain the liquid through.

Decant the elderflower lemonade into clean sterilised bottles that can be labelled and stored in the fridge.

The lemonade will keep for a couple of weeks in the fridge and can be served with a little sparkling water to pep it up.

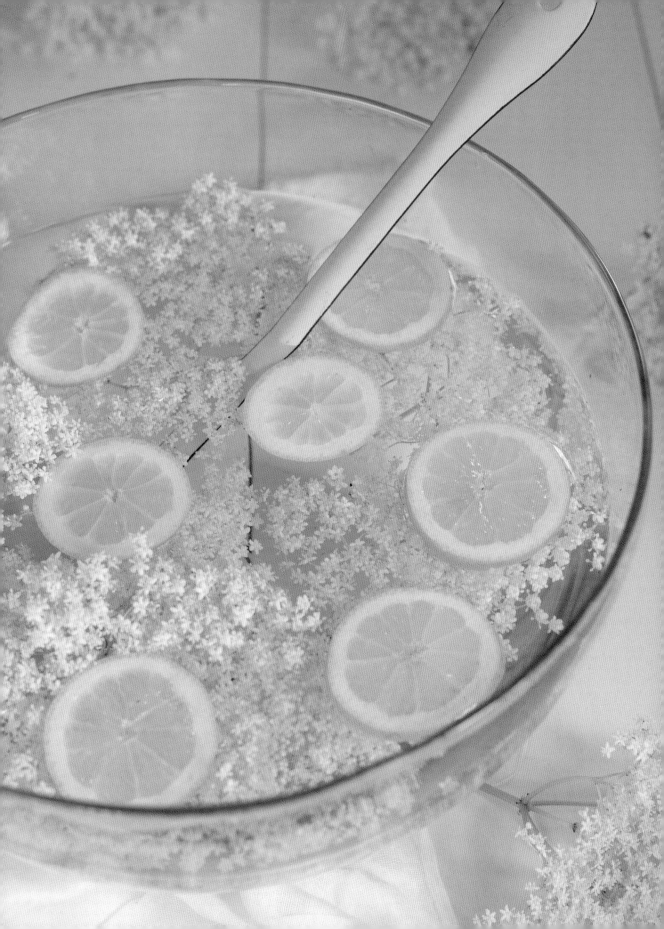

DIY HERB TEAS

Drinking herbal tea can be a solace for people with a sensitive gut. Many herbs contain naturally occurring soothing ingredients that make us feel better, rather than caffeine or other stimulants that may provoke IBS symptoms.

Herbal teas, also known as tisanes, have become a bit of a fashion statement recently, with many high-profile brands creating their own bespoke mixes of herbs in beautifully designed packaging. The only problem is they can be very expensive.

We have been experimenting and have found some easy ways of making DIY herbal teas at home for a fraction of the price charged by designer brands.

To make your own DIY tea, you can use a teapot with an in-built filter to catch the herbs as you pour. Glass pots are very attractive and look lovely filled with fresh herbs and water. Or you can buy paper tea filters, which look like empty tea bags that you fill yourself with dried or fresh herbs (see p.175). Once the bags are filled, they are used in the same way as tea bags.

Many of the fragrant, soothing herbs that can be used to make DIY herb teas are easily grown in the garden or a pot. They include:

Fennel (both fronds and seeds used)
Lemon verbena
Peppermint
Thyme

All you have to do to make a fresh herb tea is pick a bunch of herbs, rinse them, infuse them in water for 5 minutes, then strain into a cup.

Mint, liquorice root and fennel tea

Mint is a calming, refreshing herb that tastes wonderful teamed up with a few fennel fronds and liquorice. Just a small amount of liquorice root lends an almost sweet flavour to the mix. The Latin name for liquorice root is *Glycyrrhiza* (sweet root). Drugs made from liquorice root have been used to treat dyspepsia and peptic ulcers, due to their anti-inflammatory properties. The dried root is quite brittle and can be snapped into smaller pieces and then ground.

SERVES 4

Hands-on time 5 minutes

2 cm/1 in length liquorice root
a few fennel fronds or fennel bulb
   shavings
2 tsp dried mint, or a few fresh
   mint leaves
500 ml/1 pint/2 cups boiling
   water

Place the liquorice root in a mortar and grind as best as you can with a pestle; it just needs to be broken up a bit. Add the liquorice, fennel fronds and mint to a teapot and add boiling water.

Let the herbs steep for 5 minutes, then serve.

Lady Grey and orange blossom iced tea

This cool, fragrant drink can be sipped with meals. It is both refreshing and thirst-quenching. Lady Grey tea is flavoured with dried orange and lemon peel and bergamot oil.

SERVES 4

Hands-on time 5 minutes
Cooking time 5 minutes

FOR THE SUGAR SYRUP
150 g/5 oz/¾ cup caster
   (superfine) sugar
150 ml/5 fl oz/⅔ cup water

FOR THE TEA
1.5 l/2½ pints/1½ quarts water
2 Lady Grey tea bags
2 tsp orange blossom water

For the sugar syrup, place the sugar and water in a saucepan and bring to the boil. Reduce the temperature and stir to dissolve the sugar. Simmer for 3 minutes, then set aside to cool.

To make the tea, heat the water in a saucepan and add the tea bags. Turn off the heat. Remove the tea bags after 5 minutes. Add the orange blossom water, then gradually add the sugar syrup to your taste, stirring well as you do so. Decant the tea into a jug or a bottle and add the herbs and orange. Cool the tea in the fridge and serve with ice.

INDEX

Footnote references

1. Gibson, PR and Shepherd, SA (2012) *Food Choice as a Management Strategy for Irritable Bowel Syndrome. Am. J. Gastroenterology* 107: 655–666

2. Lorenz, K (1961) *King Solomon's Ring.* Transl. by Marjorie Kerr Wilson. Methuen, London.

3. Ford AC and Talley NJ (2012) *Irritable Bowel Syndrome. BMJ 2012*; 345: e5836

4. Damasio, A (1999) *The Feeling of What Happens: Body and Emotion in the Making of Consciousness.* Harcourt Brace, New York

5. Marshall, JK, Thabane, M, Garg, AX et al. (2010) *Eight Year Prognosis of Postinfectious Irritable Bowel Syndrome Following Waterborne Bacterial Dysentery. Gut* 59 (5): 605–611

6. Read, NW (2006) What Makes People Ill. *Sick and Tired: Healing the Illnesses Doctors Cannot Cure.* London. Phoenix Press. pp.26–47

7. Van der Kolk, B (2014) *The Body Keeps the Score: Brain Mind and Body in the Healing of Trauma.* Viking, New York.

8. Gibson, P (2013) Public Lecture: *Beating the Bloat: The FODMAP diet and The Irritable Bowel Syndrome.* www.med.monash.edu/cecs/gastro/education/2013-public-lecture.html

9. Francis, CY and Whorwell, PJ (1994) *Bran and Irritable Bowel Syndrome. Lancet* 344 (8914): 39–40

10. Biesiekierski, JR, Peters, SL, Newnham, ED et al. (2013) *No Effects of Gluten in Patients with Self-Reported Non-Celiac Gluten Sensitivity Following Dietary Reduction of Low-Fermentable, Poorly Absorbed, Short-Chain Carbohydrates. Gastroenterology*; 145 (2): 320–328

11. Darwin, C (1872) *The Expression of Emotion in Man and Animals.* 1965 edn. University of Chicago Press. Chicago.

12. Williams, M and Penman, D (2011) *Mindfulness: a practical guide to finding peace in a frantic world.* Piatkus, London

Stockists and suppliers

Bee pollen and liquorice root:
www.hollandandbarrett.com
Lactose-free coconut milk yogurt:
www.coyo.co.uk
Spelt and gluten-free flour and proving baskets for bread:
www.shipton-mill.com
www.dovesfarm.co.uk
Spices supplied in re-sealable pouches:
www.seasonedpioneers.co.uk
The Monash University Low-FODMAP diet App available from www.itunes.apple.com
Tea filters: www.shibui-tea.co.uk

Additional Resources

Our website:
www.cookingforthesensitivegut.com
IBS Network: www.theibsnetwork.org
For a list of Kings College London (KCL) trained FODMAP dietitians:
www.kcl.ac.uk/lsm/research/divisions/dns/projects/fodmaps/faq.aspx
The British Dietetic Association (BDA):
www.bda.uk.com
Coeliac UK: www.coeliac.org.uk
Crohn's and colitis UK:
www.crohnsandcolitis.org.uk

First published in paperback in the
United Kingdom in 2019 by
Collins & Brown
43 Great Ormond Street
London WC1N 3HZ

ISBN: 978-1-911624-10-3

A CIP catalogue record for this book is available
from the British Library.

10 9 8 7 6 5 4 3 2 1

Photographer: Joan Ransley

Reproduction by Colour Depth, UK
Printed and bound by 1010 Printing International Ltd, China

www.pavilionbooks.com

Acknowledgements

Our thanks go to our agent Michael Alcock, of Johnson and Alcock Literary Agency, for spotting the potential of this book.

Thanks also to the team at Pavilion Books for having the confidence in this project, in particular Emily Preece-Morrison and Fiona Holman, to Lucy Bannell for her assistance with editing and Laura Russell in design.

Particular thanks go to Andy Scott, a talented craftsman, for his help building the sets used in the photography, and to Michael Harris and Emma Garry Design for their valuable advice on photography and design.

Joan is particularly grateful to Natasha Byers and Lisa Jenkins for allowing her to interrupt service at their beautiful café, Toast House in Ilkley, to take photographs, and to Georgie Richmond of Toast House for being willing to be photographed.

For advice on the diet, we are grateful to Dr Jane Muir, Department of Gastoenterology, Central Clinical School, Monash University, Melbourne, Australia, for answering our questions on the latest research on FODMAPs.

Photo Credits

Emma Garry Design, fabrics and home ware
www.emmagarry.com
The Fine Cheese Company Bath for kindly
supplying tableware by John Broadley
www.finecheese.co.uk
Toast House, Leeds Road, Ilkley, West Yorkshire
www.toasthouse.co.uk